The Low-Carb
Comfort Food Cookbook

Mary Dan Eades, M.D.
Michael R. Eades, M.D.
Ursula Solom

Houghton Mifflin Harcourt
Boston   New York

To the low-carb faithful—cook well, live long.

Published by Houghton Mifflin Harcourt Publishing Company
Published simultaneously in Canada

Design and production by Navta Associates, Inc.

For information about permission to reproduce selections from this book, write to Permissions, Houghton Mifflin Harcourt Publishing Company, 215 Park Avenue South, New York, New York 10003.

www.hmhco.com

The information contained in this book is not intended to serve as a replacement for professional medical advice. Any use of the information in this book is at the reader's discretion. The author and the publisher specifically disclaim any and all liability arising directly or indirectly from the use or application of any information contained in this book. A health care professional should be consulted regarding your specific situation.

Library of Congress Cataloging-in-Publication Data:

Eades, Mary Dan.
  The low-carb comfort food cookbook / Mary Dan Eades, Michael R. Eades, Ursula Solom.
    p. cm.

  Includes bibliographical references and index.
    ISBN 0-471-26757-0 (Cloth)
    1. Cookery. 2 Low-carbohydrate diet—Recipes. I. Eades, Mary Dan.
  II. Eades, Michael R. III. Solom, Ursula. IV. Title.
  TX714 .E214 2003
  641.5'638—dc21   2002014009

Printed in the United States of America

CRNC 10 9 8 7 6 5 4

4500524350

CONTENTS

ACKNOWLEDGMENTS

No book project comes about without the help of an entire cast of people, but in this instance, we are especially indebted to the monumental contributions made by two people: Ursula Solom and Rose Crane.

Without Ursula's drive, ingenuity, creativity, energy, and never-say-die attitude as our collaborator, most of the comfort foods that you'll enjoy in this book would quite honestly not exist, they are completely her brainchild. For her tireless contribution to low-carb eating in general and to this book in particular, we are deeply grateful.

And, although she's not officially recognized on the cover, we couldn't have managed to fill the book with so many interesting recipes of all kinds without those contributed by our sister (and sister-in-law), Rose Crane, who worked for over a year to develop, modify, test, and retest many of the low-carb recipes herein. We thank her for her generosity in contributing them and her help throughout this process.

To our ever-faithful agents, Carol Mann and Channa Taub, we again say thanks for always believing in us and for once again finding the right publishing home for this project.

To our editor, Tom Miller, and all the folks at Wiley, our heartfelt thanks for recognizing the need in the marketplace for a cookbook like this one, for trimming it and shaping it into its final form, and for making this idea a reality for all of us.

Thanks to our overworked assistant, Kristi McAfee, for putting up with our hectic lives, wading through piles of papers, fielding phone calls, faxing, mailing, emailing, and chauffeuring at all hours of the day and night—what would we ever do without you?

And, finally, our appreciation and love go to our immediate family: our sons, Ted, Dan, and Scott; their wives, Jamye and Katherine; and our grandsons, Thomas and William, for always loving us, laughing with us, believing in us, and giving us the best seven reasons of all to keep doing what we do.

Michael and Mary Dan Eades

*****

Two individuals stand out in particular because of the special influence they had over shaping this book. Without them, my low-carb comfort food recipes might never have seen the light of day. First and foremost, there is Richard K. Bernstein, M.D., the renowned physician and diabetologist in Mamaroneck, New York. I am thankful and grateful beyond measure for the interest he took in my fledgling efforts, when I, a total stranger, approached him. he took the time to read, review, counsel—and in the end gave my project a resounding thumbs up. He introduced me to his literary agent, Channa Taub, who became the other moving force in this venture, because she, too, quickly became a believer. When Channa first asked me to send her what I had, she minced no words about what she wanted. She was not looking for diet manuals or "more ways to fix chicken"; she was only interested in *original* low-carb recipes, for they were badly needed. If I truly had those, she might consider representing me. Once won over, Channa's unwavering belief in what she thought I could accomplish often helped bolster my own, at times flagging, self-confidence when faced with tough problems. She was always there, patiently guiding and advising. Her vision of the book tremendously broadened its original focus and scope, making it far better. She also initiated the collaboration with the Drs. Eades. I owe Channa a huge debt of gratitude for accepting me and for putting her trust in me.

Heartfelt thanks and admiration also go to my other agent, Carol Mann, who worked diligently and brilliantly to place this book with a great publishing house and a terrific editor, Tom Miller. As appears to be true of all the people involved with this book, he, too, had an infectious enthusiasm for it and believed in its importance and success from the outset. He decided to put the book on a fast track to bring it out quickly. For him, it meant working tirelessly, despite an already enormous workload. He trimmed, shaped, and streamlined the manuscript into the fabulous, sleek volume you hold in your hands, one that will make it a joy to cook low-carb. I cannot thank him enough.

When the Drs. Eades and I reached agreement on a collaboration, we all expected that the result would be a wonderful cookbook, one that would be far better than any two books we might have published separately could have been. But what would it be like working with them? What can I say, except that, in just one respect, I regret the project has now ended. I could not have asked for nicer or better partners and shall greatly miss working with them. Mike and Mary Dan rolled up their sleeves and pitched in to do whatever needed doing. They did it with a sense of humor, through thick and thin, through hairy deadlines and other minor calamities of publishing. They also gave me many good ideas and suggestions to make the book even more useful and interesting. If my recipes should help to make this incredibly powerful diet more user friendly, thus enabling many more people than before to make a long-term commitment to it and take advantage of this marvelous way to lose weight and usually also gain other, significant health benefits, I would consider it a tiny payback for what the Drs. Eades truly have done for me, personally—and of which I am reminded every single day: they restored my health. Words can hardly say it properly, but I thank them from the bottom of my heart.

It wasn't until the first successful Magic Rolls came off the cookie sheet that I knew the tide was turning. This had not happened at the usual tidal speed, however, but only after a long interval that saw literally thousands of hopeless specimens go down the drain. No one stood closer and remained more supportive and optimistic than my husband, Bob, who might rightly have asked if I really thought anything would ever come of what I was trying to do. I cannot thank him enough for his unfaltering support, his love, his honest judgment, and his highly critical taste buds that often sent me flying back to the drawing board. He kept the project or, rather, me, on track—not always a small feat. It would have taken far longer to complete the book if it had not been for him.

Finally, thanks to my three daughters, Karen, Sandra, and Hilary, who were supportive and always convinced that their mom could pull this off. They also constantly reminded me of the need to keep the recipes easy and quick to make, useful for busy lives. Thanks, too, go to my brother-in-law, Donald Solom, who helped with the testing of recipes, and to my brother, Dr. Guenther Patzig, whose sage counsel and sometimes irreverent sense of humor never failed to lighten a task.

Ursula Solom

INTRODUCTION

It's clear that low-carb dieting is here to stay. It is estimated that 25 million North Americans have followed or currently follow some variation of the low-carb nutritional theme—for example, our own Protein Power Plan, Dr. Atkins, SugarBusters!, the Carbohydrate Addicts Diet, the Zone, the Paleo Diet, Suzanne Somers, or another low-carb diet. And from the ranks of this vast multitude of low-carb devotees has come an avalanche of letters, postcards, emails, faxes, and phone calls with a strong recurring theme: give us more recipes, quicker meal plans, and budget-minded ideas for sticking to low carb forever.

In response to that need, we (Mary Dan and Michael Eades) set to work accumulating and testing low-carb recipes for tasty dishes that would be quick and easy to prepare and wouldn't bust the budget at the grocery store checkout. We accumulated some great recipes for traditional low-carb staples (meats, fish, poultry, eggs, cheese, and low-starch fruits and vegetables), along with menu ideas and preparation instructions to help low-carb dieters entertain friends and family at the many feasting celebrations that occur throughout the year. We were on track to produce a traditional cookbook that we thought would help our readers live low carb more easily. Then, as is so often the case, Serendipity, that shy muse of fortuitous coincidence, intervened in the form of a call from our agent, Channa Taub.

She had recently accepted a new client who was working on a low-carb cookbook with intriguing and unusual recipes. Channa felt that a collaboration between us might yield some exciting results. And so it was that we first met Ursula Solom.

When we first spoke with Ursula by phone, we realized she was industrious and intrepid. She had spent many years in Alaska as a bio-medical research librarian and later, as library director, developed the fledgling Alaska Health Sciences Library into an institution that pro-vides statewide medical library services to health professionals. Then, having conquered that realm, she picked another frontier with a move to Hawaii to develop a macadamia nut farm—planting and tending the trees with her own hands. We were amazed by her grit and ability.

And so it was that we traveled to Spokane, Washington, to meet Ursula and to view firsthand what she claimed to have hit upon. She had spent two years doing research of her own, developing recipes for a low-carb cookbook that included many foods previously forbidden on low-carb eating plans. She had arrived at an ingenious way to make protein and fats behave like starches in baking—a low-carb nirvana.

We worked together in her test kitchen as she showed us how to prepare these recipes. There were raised-yeast breads and rolls, hearty peasant breads, a half-dozen different muffins and sweet breads, and biscuits that tasted too good to be low carb. She showed us coffee cakes, streusel, and banana bread warm from the oven, topped with creamy butter. She could turn out waffles and pancakes so light and delicate you'd swear they were the real thing. She'd even figured out ways to make piecrust, focaccia, tortillas, and pizza dough. And the pièce de résistance . . . pasta! We knew that in collaboration the three of us could develop not just a good low-carb cookbook but a partner-ship that would bring low-carb devotees something they'd missed: comfort foods in perfect sync with their commitment to low-carb eating.

You'll hear two distinct voices in this book. Those readers familiar with our previous works, *Protein Power* and the *Protein Power Life Plan*, will recognize our Southern touch in the text of many of the recipes, introductions to chapters, and elsewhere. The other voice belongs to Ursula, and you'll quickly come to recognize it, too.

For a low-carb dieter, this book is a godsend. Now you'll be able to indulge in all those guilty pleasures you used to reserve for dietary vacations: apple pie à la mode, Danish pastries, spaghetti and meat-balls, garlic bread, toast, waffles, muffins, brownies, pound cake . . . even pizza. It's all back on the table for the devoted low-carber. Now, you really can have your cake and eat it too.

You'll find this cookbook arranged in the order that you would eat throughout the day. It begins with bread, because who hasn't missed bread on a low-carb plan? Then it moves to the other things you'd like to have for breakfast. If you've been low-carbing long, you'll appreciate having delicious recipes for waffles, pancakes, and crepes. Then it's on to lunches and dinners, organized as you'd expect to see them on a menu: appetizers, soups, salads, entrees of every description, and sweets.

You'll be amazed at the variety of entrees—many dishes you thought you'd never see on a low-carb menu. For example, have you missed having Italian food on a low-carb plan? Well, prepare yourself for lasagna and garlic bread again. You'll find recipes for real, honest-to-goodness pasta. That means beef Stroganoff, too. And it's goodbye to eating just the toppings off the pizza—now you can have crust and all. Or maybe it's Mexican food that you're longing for. There are enchiladas, nachos, fajitas, even refried beans and low-carb "pasta rice," all without the heavy carb cost that's kept you from eating them—or made you suffer pangs of guilt if you did.

In the dessert department, you'll once again be able to enjoy your favorite cookies, cakes, pies, shortcake, ice cream, and chocolate truffles without regret and still keep your low-carb commitment to good health and fitness. And what's more, many of these delicious recipes for breads, cookies, and muffins are not only low in carbohydrates, but they're gluten-free, too, making them suitable for a large segment of readers who suffer both from insulin resistance disorders, requiring a low-carbohydrate regimen, and intolerance to wheat, making even a sandwich off limits. Previously, these people had a choice to make: eat high-carb gluten-free products if they desired a bit of bread or cake, or simply miss out. *The Low-Carb Comfort Food Cookbook* fills both needs. So let them eat cake!

We—all three of us—hope that by using this book you'll learn to love living your low-carb life every day and that our collaboration will make it easier for you to stick to your low-carb plan no matter what occasion may arise. It's our wish that within these covers you'll find everything you need to eat well and live long. *Buon appetito!*

1

LOW-CARB COMFORT FOOD COOKING GUIDELINES

LOW-CARB INGREDIENTS

Low-carb cooking used to be mostly a matter of deprivation and restrictions. That was its main impact on the low-carb kitchen. You could not eat *this;* you could not eat *that.* It made cooking and eating boring but also fairly simple. Foods with high-carbohydrate concentrations were largely out. It is one thing to understand that you do not really need to eat much, if any, carbohydrate-laden foods to be healthy and quite another to live by that rule. No hearty sandwiches, no dinner rolls, no hamburger buns, no muffins, not to mention pasta, pizza, and tortillas. Well, now you are released from these restrictions. With the recipes you will find here, you can eat almost anything you have been missing (at least within reason) and still control your weight and maintain a great lipid profile. It's obviously not because carbohydrate foods are okay again; it is simply that in this cookbook your favorite foods are made to appear rich in carbs, even though the actual carb counts are quite low or kept to a tolerable minimum. And none of it happens at the expense of taste.

How do we do it? By eliminating the worst offenders, which are the starchy, high-carb grains (and all products made from them) along with that pure carbohydrate, sugar. Both must be exiled, except for small amounts. And that is all there is to it. Less simple, of course, is what to do about it. It has taken years to find substitutes for flour and sugar to create these workable recipes. Of the two, the sugar problem has been the easier one to deal with. Today, some acceptable artificial sweeteners that can also be used in baking are available and generally work fine. On occasion—when texture truly demands it—limited amounts of real sugar can be added to a recipe as well. (Sweeteners are discussed later in this chapter.)

The chief difficulty is finding a replacement for flour. What breads, cookies, rolls, crackers, cereal, pancakes, muffins, pizza, or pasta can you make without it? None, obviously. Flour supplies the bulk in all of these beloved foods. But at 92.0 grams of carb in a single cup of white flour and only slightly fewer in a cup of whole-wheat flour, *flour is the number one enemy of the low-carb dieter.* So the principal change in your new low-carb kitchen will revolve around what can be used in its place. Everything else remains pretty much the same.

Flour—that powdery, tasteless, valuable stuff—has no perfect match for baking. Impostors are hard to find. There are, however, substances that collectively can do a pretty good job of imitating the texture that comes from flour, and that's what we are after. So instead of using flour, you will be using one or more of these different ingredients. Piling these items into the mixing bowl to make a batch of bread, muffins, or rolls will quickly become routine.

Some of these new flour substitutes may already be familiar to you. The main ones are (1) *almonds*—usually ground into a meal or flour; (2) *vital wheat gluten flour*—a flour with most of the starch removed; (3) *wheat bran*—known to most of us as a good source of fiber, a flaky meal made from the outer layer or husk of the wheat kernel; (4) *whey protein powder*—a powdery substance made from the watery part of milk; and (5) *soy protein powder*—a powdery substance like whey protein but extracted from the soybean. These ingredients will help to make you believe that you are eating flour. You can usually find them in the health food section of your supermarket or in most health food stores. Prices vary, so you will want to comparison shop for the best deals. You also have the option to order all the items you need from one single source at fabulous prices and have them delivered directly to your door (see "Mail-Order Sources"). Let's check out the individual low-carb magicians.

LOW-CARB FLOUR PRETENDERS

Almonds

The almond is an excellent flour replacer. It is rich in monounsaturated oils, vitamin E, calcium, magnesium, potassium, and other beneficial nutrients but light on carbs. Ground almonds have just 3.0 grams of carb in ¼ cup. By contrast, ¼ cup of white flour has 23.0 grams and is close to a nutritional zero. With a food processor or good blender, it's easy to grind the nuts to a uniform meal. However, you can simply purchase a ready-made flour or meal made from whole or blanched almonds. (Never buy defatted or partially defatted meals or flours.) Most recipes call for whole almond meal. Blanched almond flour has a lighter texture and can be used interchangeably. Unlike whole nuts, which you can get in many places, you might need to order the meal. We have found it at prices that are likely to be lower than that of whole nuts you buy locally (see "Mail-Order Sources").

Vital Wheat Gluten Flour

Think of this flour as the reverse of white flour, which is what it is. Regular white flour has 23.0 grams of carb in ¼ cup. Vital wheat gluten flour, in contrast, has just 5.6 grams of carb in ¼ cup. Also, white flour has 3.0 grams of protein in ¼ cup, whereas vital wheat gluten has 26.0 grams. Vital wheat gluten flour looks and feels a lot like flour, which makes it exceptionally handy in baking.

Some folks have an allergy to *gluten,* the name given to certain proteins found in wheat, rye, barley, and oats. Affected individuals cannot eat foods containing gluten. This takes wheat and the other grains off the table for them. Fortunately, there are many gluten-free recipes in this book—waffles, pancakes, crepes, certain quick breads, cookies, bread crumbs, croutons, and more. So if you happen to have this problem, it will still be possible for you to enjoy many low-carb treats.

Unprocessed (crude) Wheat Bran

You know it as a good source of fiber, but wheat bran is also low in carbs. There are 3.0 grams of carb, 2.0 grams of protein, and 6.0 grams of fiber in ¼ cup of crude wheat bran, so it is helpful in many ways, especially in replacing the bulk that comes from traditional flours in baking. When you buy crude wheat bran, especially in bulk quantities, make sure it is not stale—it should have almost no smell. You can improve the flavor of bran slightly by toasting it. Just put 3 or 4 cups in a large, shallow baking pan and toast the bran for about 25 to 30 minutes at 300°F. You can also buy Kretschmer's Toasted Wheat Bran, which is ready to go.

Whey Protein Powder

Whey protein powder appears in the recipes here in small amounts and mainly for its terrific value as a usable protein and its beneficial effect on the immune system. Baked goods made with it tend to be slightly fragile or delicate, and as a practical matter, whey does not work quite as well as some other products in replacing flour. In health food stores, you will usually find whey protein next to soy protein powder and other proteins. Look for a whey powder that says it is ultra- or microfiltered. It comes in several flavors as well as plain. For cooking and baking it's best to use plain (natural or unflavored) whey to avoid adding unintended flavors. Whey protein can also become the base for terrific high-protein shakes and smoothies that make wonderful power breakfasts (or anytime meals). For that purpose, choose from the fun flavors—chocolate, vanilla, strawberry, mocha— you can purchase besides the plain variety. Or, if you like, you can simply add flavor to the natural whey with fresh or frozen fruits or flavor extracts. The carb count for whey protein varies with the product, so check labels when you buy it. In this cookbook we have assigned whey an average value of 3.0 grams of carb per ¼ cup (about 1 ounce) and 20.0 grams of protein for the same amount.

Soy Protein Powder

Unlike whey protein, pure soy protein powder has no carbs. It has both a neutral flavor and a texture that make it useful as a flour substitute. It is extremely helpful in low-carb cooking. If you want to reduce carbs dramatically, soy protein powder is the ingredient of choice. Soy protein powder is used in many commercial soy-based foods.

Some newer research suggests that the manufacturing processes used to make these *soy protein isolates* (found not only in soy protein powders but in some forms of tofu, soy milk products, texturized vegetable protein, and other soy products) may damage the proteins and produce possibly harmful substances. Despite its growing reputation as a health food—and there certainly seems to be some evidence for health benefits from naturally fermented soy products in certain conditions—the jury is still out on the health benefits, or, more importantly, the health risks of eating large amounts of processed soy. Until more definitive information becomes available, soy protein powder is used slightly more sparingly in the recipes in this book than it might have been otherwise. Since soy protein powder is never the main ingredient in any recipe, you will not be eating large amounts. If the use of processed soy concerns you, however, you can substitute whey protein powder for soy protein powder in a ratio of ⅓ cup whey protein powder for every ¼ cup of soy protein powder, with a slight gain in carb, and, depending on the whey protein you use, a slight loss in texture.

Another choice is to substitute equal amounts of soy protein powder with equal amounts of full-fat roasted or full-fat raw *soy flour.* Soy flour has 5.5 grams of carb in ¼ cup and 7.4 grams of protein.

Unlike soy protein powder, it has a pronounced flavor, which will come through if you use the flour in all but small amounts. Not everyone likes this particular taste. Soy flour is available in most health food stores and in many supermarkets.

Black Soybeans

The black soybean is not much of a flour substitute, but it possesses marvelous and unusual qualities. Unlike its cousins, black beans, garbanzo beans, navy beans, kidney beans, and so on, which weigh in at about 20.0 grams of carb in ½ cup and are pretty nearly off limits on a low-carb diet, this precious little legume has only 3.2 grams of carb, 6.9 grams of protein, and 3.8 grams of fiber in ½ cup. Black soybeans will help satisfy your craving for the legumes you cannot eat or can eat only sparingly. Beyond doing "bean duty," though, the black soybean's fairly neutral flavor and mealy texture makes it useful in unexpected places, even in some cookies and candies. The beans also come in quite handy as an unobtrusive thickener. Black soybeans (Eden Organic Soybeans and Shari's, to name two brands) are available in most health food stores and many supermarkets.

SWEETENERS

Before you read anything about sweeteners—natural or artificial—bear in mind that the best course of all is to use sweeteners *as little as possible*. Less really is better.

"Beat butter and sugar until thick and creamy; add eggs, one at a time"—how many great cookie recipes begin this way? The result is cookies with a divine texture. Well, you can never follow that dictate again. That cup of sugar you are asked to add to the butter in traditional cookie recipes clocks in at 198.0 grams of carb. But do not feel too disappointed. With just a few exceptions, you can mimic the sugar–butter–egg combo successfully with the recipes here. Only the rare recipe needs a small boost from real sugar. Most of the time the substitute sweetener works well—and does so for just a fraction of the carb cost of real sugar.

Splenda

Artificial sweeteners that you can use not only in beverages but also in *cooking* and *baking*—sweeteners that taste good, do not deteriorate in heat, and are not, at this time, known to be harmful—are limited. The sweetener of choice in this book is sucralose (trade name: Splenda)[1]. It has been around for over a decade in several countries,

---

[1] We do not recommend the use of aspartame because: 1. Research has suggested that it may be harmful to the brain, and 2. It doesn't hold up to cooking temperatures.

including Canada, and received FDA approval in the United States in 2000. Sucralose is made from table sugar that has been chemically and ingeniously altered so that your body has no idea that this is sugar and thus allows it to pass through with insulin asleep at the switch. You, on the other hand, can enjoy the pleasant sweetening powers it possesses. Still, there are drawbacks.

The compound is said to be 600 times sweeter than the sugar from which it is derived. To make it a substance—one that is visible, that is—it needs to be packed with a carrier. At the time of this writing, you can buy Splenda (in the United States) as small packets or as a granular powder that can be used as if it were real sugar. Both forms are available in most supermarkets. The bulking or carrying agents for Splenda are maltodextrin and dextrose. They are what you "see" when you open a box or packet. Both are sugars. This diminishes the effect of the sugar-free sucralose. Two teaspoons of the loose powder (or one packet, the equivalent of 2 teaspoons) contain 1.0 gram of carb or a bit less. Count either as 1.0 gram. In subjective taste tests—you can do this yourself—the packets appear to sweeten a little better than equivalent amounts of the granular powder. So the recipes in this book suggest using Splenda packets, but feel free to use the granular form. You can reduce or increase the amount of sweetener in any recipe. Use as little as needed to satisfy your taste buds. (As a reference point, a cup of sugar is equivalent to about 24 packets of Splenda.)

The sweetener is also manufactured in tablet form in 200-count dispensers (like the Equal tablets that are made from aspartame). Tablets are superior to other forms of the Splenda sweetener because the pills carry little in the way of bulk. Ten tablets equal 5 packets of Splenda and have only 1.0 gram of carb. They are easy to crush to a powder with a mortar and pestle. The downside is that the tablets are not currently available in the United States. It is to be hoped that this will change. You may want to check the www.Splenda.com website or the Drs. Eades's website, www.eatprotein.com, for new information on tablet availability.

Stevia

Although not featured in recipes in this book, you can substitute other sweeteners. One is stevia, a product coaxed from the leaves of the *Stevia rebaudiana* plant and sold as a bulk powder, in packets, or as a liquid in health food stores. The compound isn't advertised as a sweetener, because, despite its safety and potent sweetness, the Food and Drug Administration hasn't given permission for this product to be labeled as such. Look for it alongside vitamin supplements instead of with the sugars. Stevia is stable in liquids, heat-stable for baking, and appears to have little effect on blood sugar. It can be a useful addition to the low-carb kitchen, but be cautious with it; if you use too much, it tends to taste bitter.

Sugar Alcohols

Nature also makes substances known as sugar alcohols. They taste sweet, but, curiously, are not readily absorbed into the blood and thus cannot alert your body's insulin patrol. You'll recognize their names—sorbitol, mannitol, maltitol, and xylitol—from the labels of many sugar-free products. You can also buy them separately to use in cooking and baking. Although they may sound great, they come with one important disadvantage. Since they're not absorbed, eating too much of them is likely going to give you diarrhea. Products made with these sweeteners always carry this warning. You will quickly know when you have eaten more than you should.

Real Sugars

What if you do not want to use any artificial sweeteners? Use exceedingly small doses of table sugar or honey, instead. Even small amounts, however, will catapult you into much higher brackets of carb. Two teaspoons of real table sugar have 8.0 grams of carb; 2 teaspoons of honey have 11.3 grams—as opposed to the 1.0 gram in a packet (2 teaspoons) of Splenda.

It's good to keep in mind—and easy to forget—that no matter which sweetener you pick, sugary things are part of this cookbook not because you need them—you don't—but because you love them and miss them and cannot seem to get along without them. Having them available with very few carbs should help you to stay away from the "real stuff" and to stick to your commitment to good health and fitness. Just remember this: *Always exercise restraint.*

LOW-CARB COMFORT FOOD, LOSING WEIGHT, AND YOUR HEALTH

Unlike many other cookbooks, this book allows you to see at a glance how many grams of carb and protein are in every single ingredient in a recipe. The counts almost always appear next to each food entry. You can also see what the total carb and protein counts are for a recipe as well as for individual servings. The reason for this arrangement is to help you keep close track of the carb you eat and to see to it that you get enough protein in your diet.

As you know, you need not count calories. The marching orders are quite simple: *eat only until you are satisfied and never, never,*

never stuff yourself. Adhere to this basic rule and you should be successful with your diet.

A word of caution is important here. The recipes in this book are geared to low-carb comfort food that should keep you happy and satisfied—food that will help you stay on the diet. While these recipes are low in carbs, they are not necessarily low in calories. Many make liberal use of eggs, cream cheese, cream, butter, olive oil, and nuts to mimic the texture and bulk of the flour you have to give up. If you are still in the weight-reduction phase of your eating regimen, you could stall your weight loss by eating too many servings of such delights as low-carb pasta, breads, waffles, and muffins. The same is true for most desserts; custard, for instance, is mainly eggs and heavy cream. Although you can still lower triglycerides and cholesterol, drop blood pressure, and stabilize blood sugar if you overeat these low-carb treats, you will not lose weight as effectively. To lose weight, you must create a calorie deficit—fewer calories coming in than your body needs to fuel itself. Use these delicious recipes with a dose of common sense during your weight loss to keep your diet interesting—and comforting—and to keep you on the low-carb track.

After you have reached your weight goal, you can enjoy these wonderful foods in much greater amounts and still maintain your loss. As long as you understand these limitations, your main job is to be vigilant about carbs. On the *Protein Power* plan, we recommend a carbohydrate intake of 10 to 15 effective grams per meal or snack (three meals and one snack per day) during the *Intervention* phase when you're reducing your weight and/or correcting health problems. Once that's achieved, we ask that you progress to *Transition,* increasing your carb intake per meal to 15 to 25 effective grams for a few weeks, then move on to *Maintenance,* where you can enjoy 25 to 30 grams per meal or more depending on your personal ability to tolerate carbs. The amount of carbohydrate tolerated in the maintenance phase will vary from person to person. The goal in maintenance is to stick to a daily count that allows you to maintain your weight and your control of any health issues, such as elevated blood pressure, high blood sugar, or high blood cholesterol or triglyceride levels. If you see those start to slip away, reduce your carb allotment to the transition level (or if things have really gotten away from you, to the intervention level) until you regain control again.

Another issue that bears mention is the effect on weight loss of excess calorie intake, although for most people on a low-carb diet, such as the *Protein Power* plan, calories play a minor role; just controlling carb intake is sufficient to restore health and reduce excess weight. Other people, however, need to be more mindful of both how many calories and how many carbs they eat. This caution applies primarily to people who are of smaller stature or who don't have a tremendous amount of weight to lose. If you are still in the weight-loss phase of your diet and your progress stalls, the first concern is that you're eating too many calories. If your body is meeting all its energy needs from the food you're eating—even if it's low-carb food—it has no reason to turn to its fat stores. Because many of the low-carb treats in this cookbook are dense in calories, eating them with reckless abandon—even within your carb limit—might stall your loss. And although the health benefits of low-carb eating aren't particularly affected by calories, weight loss can be. If you stall your progress in losing weight, look to see if you're treating yourself too often to too many of these low-carb comfort pleasures and cut back your intake somewhat until your weight loss resumes. Once you reach maintenance, calorie intake doesn't matter as much and you can enjoy more of them.

Whatever your personal carb allotment, stick to it or even below it. The carb counts given for individual ingredients are meant to encourage you to be watchful of your intake; they will also help you recalculate the numbers if you want to double or reduce a particular recipe or make other changes.

In nutritional lingo, the standard abbreviation for carbohydrate is CHO and for protein it is PRO. We've stuck to these abbreviations in this book. Where do the numbers come from? There are several sources: *The Protein Power LifePlan Gram Counter,* by Michael R. Eades, M.D., and Mary Dan Eades, M.D.; *The Complete Book of Food Counts,* by Corinne T. Netzer; *Bowes & Church's Food Values of Portions Commonly Used* (17th ed.), by J. A. Pennington; and the ESHA Research nutritional database files. You may notice occasional, slight discrepancies in the gram counts. Food samples being analyzed by different organizations may have slightly different characteristics based on a variety of conditions, such as ripeness and water content, so carb counts can vary from source to source. While 100 percent accuracy may remain elusive, the numbers are close; use them as a guide. If you are under severe carbohydrate restrictions, you may want to add 10 percent across the board to all total carb counts just to build in a little cushion.

Besides the slight discrepancies in carb counts, there is another little problem that can lead to a bit of confusion—the way carb grams are sometimes counted. The ubiquitous nutrition fact labels give counts for total carbohydrates, which include fiber. Fiber is also listed separately as a subheading of total carbs. Although fiber is a carbohydrate, it is indigestible by humans. It just passes through, pretty much unchanged, without having a carbohydrate impact; therefore, it does not count. You can deduct this amount from the total carb counts on nutrition labels. This confusing situation gave rise to a new concept, coined by the Drs. Eades, and called effective carbohydrate content or ECC. The term originated in the bestseller *Protein Power* and was expanded in *The Protein Power LifePlan*. The ECC represents the grams of carbohydrate present in a food as sugar or starch *with the fiber already deducted*. The counts in this book are based on the ECC and so are the numbers in *The Protein Power LifePlan* and *The Protein Power LifePlan Gram Counter*.

FATS

Fats will have an impact on your low-carb program in the sense that you can use them more freely than you may have done in the past. In these recipes you will be using such fats as butter, olive oil, coconut oil, cream cheese, cream, and eggs in greater quantities than you may have previously. Properly handled, these fats can exert a beneficial effect on your health.

Trans Fats

You will want to avoid certain other fats. You'll find these in fats commonly used in cooking, such as margarine, vegetable shortening, and vegetable oils (soybean oil, corn oil, sunflower oil, safflower oil, and others). These fats or oils have been altered by the manufacturer (through application of chemicals, heat, and pressure) to make them more shelf-stable. The process damages the oils, creating substances called *trans fats,* which have been proven to promote heart disease and possibly even diabetes and certain cancers. Today, you see some margarines on store shelves that proclaim to contain no *trans* fats and you may be tempted to use them. However, as of this writing, the jury is still out about how the manufacturer has stabilized the vegetable oils without creating *trans* fats and whether these margarines are truly safe to use, so we do not encourage their use in cooking. Avoiding *trans* fats is usually easy. The clue to their presence is found in two words that show up on most labels of fats or oils that harbor them: *partially hydrogenated.* When you see them, avoid the product. Be aware, however, that not all labels will be so forthcoming, listing only "vegetable oil" or "soybean oil," either of which is likely to contain *trans* fats.

Canola Oil

Canola oil is often touted as a healthy oil because it contains large amounts of monounsaturated fat, like olive oil. Unfortunately, processing methods damage it. In its natural state, canola oil has a strong and unpalatable odor. The deodorizing methods currently employed to remove these unpleasant characteristics also cause the formation of *trans* fats, even in cold-pressed canola oils and products (such as mayonnaise and salad dressings) made from them. For this reason, we discourage the use of canola oil.

Flaxseed Oil

Flaxseed oil is a highly delicate oil with a strong and distinctive odor that must be removed to make it commercially acceptable. Because of the high percentage of alpha-linolenic acid in flaxseed oil, just like canola oil, it can also be damaged in the deodorizing process, turning an otherwise wonderful oil into a bottle of *trans* fats. If you're a devotee of the health benefits of the delicate and beneficial oils found in flaxseeds, grind the seeds fresh in small amounts to add to salads and shakes. Never heat flaxseed. Discard it promptly if it turns the least bit rancid.

Good Fats

Acceptable oils are usually cold-extracted (cold-pressed) and have no added chemicals in them. Labels tell you this, too. The first extraction preserves the full amount of vitamins; subsequent extractions of oils are less rich and have less flavor, but this is not necessarily a bad thing. The oils of the first extraction (the most expensive ones as a rule) are labeled "extra virgin," with varying lesser grades of perfection found among the oils of subsequent pressings or extractions. Reserve high-quality oils to eat unadulterated—for dipping focaccia, on salads, drizzled over tomatoes—or when you have a recipe that really demands a strong, rich taste. Besides extra virgin olive oil, you might want to keep some small bottles of nut oils (walnut, cashew, macadamia, sesame) on hand and try them out, too. All of these oils can be stored at room temperature if you use them regularly but should be protected from light. Experiment a little with the different tastes of these oils. It's fun.

For baking and lower-temperature cooking, you can or might want to use lighter, less flavorful grades of oil. There is one caveat that requires you to read labels again: lighter oils, including lighter grades of olive oils, can sometimes be mixtures of oils. The added oils are not necessarily cold-extracted and could be a potential source of *trans* fats. The presence of partially hydrogenated fats is supposed to be stated on the label; this is not always the case, however, notably with soybean oil, so beware.

For frying you must use oils that hold up well under high temperatures. In this book we frequently use coconut oil. It remains heat-stable during cooking and tolerates the most heat before reaching the smoking point. It's great for baking, too, in place of butter, shortening, or lard, and can be used interchangeably with these fats in most cooking. As with all good oils, coconut oil should be a natural product, either expeller-pressed or cold-pressed. Coconut oil is heavily saturated, which makes it solid at room temperature, though it quickly melts at temperatures even a few degrees higher. You can find coconut oil in some supermarkets and health food stores alongside the olive oil and other oils, but since it is solid, it is packaged in a mayonnaise-like jar. Being highly saturated, coconut and other tropical oils have earned an undeserved bad reputation as unhealthy oils. Nothing could be further from the truth. In fact, the high lauric acid content of coconut oil (one of the important fats found in human breast milk) has been shown to have antiinfective properties, so you may use it in good conscience and good health.

If you are still using margarine, replace it with butter. Butter is a wonderful spread and useful for cooking and baking as well. The best butter to buy is organic. It does not contain antibiotics, pesticides, hormones, or other chemicals. Even lard is okay to use if it is natural, not processed, and of good quality, as is fat contained in poultry or beef. The one caveat, however, is that the healthy quality of animal fats is only as good as the animal itself. Healthier fat comes from animals that have been naturally raised (without hormones, antibiotics, or pesticides).

FATS FOR COOKING AND LOW-TEMPERATURE PANFRYING

Butter
Ghee (clarified butter)
Olive oil
Coconut oil (natural)
Sesame seed oil
Lard (natural)
Fats found in naturally raised meats and poultry

FATS FOR BAKING AND FRYING

Butter
Ghee
Coconut oil
Olive oil
Lard

OILS FOR SALADS

Avocado oil
Almond oil
Cashew nut oil
Hazelnut oil
Macadamia nut oil
Olive oil
Peanut oil
Sesame seed oil
Walnut oil

Now you know what the ingredients are that will allow you—truly with just minimal effort—to make a big change in your low-carb diet and life. You can eat *seemingly* high-carb foods. And once you get used to the new routine, eating will become as normal as it always has been. Suddenly you can have it all. You are ready to go for it.

The *Protein Power* diet is not a magic gimmick; there are good, sound reasons for its tremendous success. So if the diet is new for you or you continue to have questions about the how and why of low-carb dieting, pick up a copy of *The Protein Power LifePlan* for all the answers and the newest research about living a long and healthy low-carb life.

2

BREAD AND OTHER DELICIOUS LOW-CARB BAKED GOODS

If the low-carb diet has worked miracles for you, you probably feel that it is a lifesaver. Maybe, like millions of others, you've lost a substantial amount of weight or solved difficult health problems, such as elevated cholesterol, triglycerides, or blood sugar, courtesy of the low-carb approach. And yet, in spite of its great effectiveness, low-carb devotees sometimes do fall off the plan, revert to old habits, and often see their health and weight goals begin to slip from their grasp. What could make a person stray from such success? The answer won't surprise you—in a word, *bread*. A chewy roll, a warm muffin, a fragrant cinnamon bun—who doesn't love them? And what committed low-carb dieter doesn't miss them?

Well, now we can celebrate together. Bread is back in a nutritious, guilt-free form, perfectly in sync with a low-carb diet. In this chapter, you'll find a full basket of it, with dozens of recipes for delicious, low-carb, high-protein breads, pastries, and muffins that are practically a full meal by themselves. With just a little time and even less practice—even a novice baker can follow these easy recipes—the smell of freshly baked bread will once again fill your kitchen. You'll be whipping up quick breads, dinner rolls, and home-baked biscuits and muffins even if you've never baked bread before. Got 15 minutes to spare on a Saturday? Then you've got the time to stir up the dough to make a couple of loaves of sourdough, whole-wheat, or gourmet rye bread, or almost no-carb bread. How about a batch of cinnamon buns for a quick high-protein breakfast on the run? Call your friends and tell them the Saturday morning coffee klatch is back on.

Magic Rolls

Heat water and butter, pour in a mix of vital wheat gluten flour and white flour, and stir until the mixture is a smooth mass (it takes just seconds). Beat in eggs and place the dough on a cookie sheet. This effort takes 15 minutes. The feather-light rolls that have a slight crunch to the crust and a fluffy, chewy interior will be in the oven baking. You can make them in different sizes to suit your needs. The basic recipe gives eighteen 3½ inch rolls at 2.8 grams of carb each and 5.8 grams of protein. Whatever size you make, directions are the same. The rolls freeze superbly—just remove them from bag for thawing and eat. If you are in a hurry, you can speed up the thawing process in a hot oven. No time to sit down for breakfast? Walk out with butter and cream cheese on a roll or two (replacing that hopelessly high-carb bagel). A fried egg and a slice of ham on a roll are great.

Never throw rolls away! Save them for making the best bread crumbs to be used in many recipes in this book. These rolls fit on a 13 × 17-inch cookie sheet. Use a heavy-gauge metal nonstick cookie sheet. Bake all rolls at one time. Do not grease sheet. The rolls should not stick. If they ever do, replace cookie sheet.

Choose how many rolls you want to make (18, 16, or 12) and follow these directions. Carb and protein counts for each roll appear with the serving size.

PREPARATION TIME: 15 minutes. BAKING TIME: 25 to 28 minutes.
SERVING SIZE: one roll (of 18). AMOUNT PER SERVING: 2.8 grams of carb, 5.8 grams of protein.
SERVING SIZE: one roll (of 16). AMOUNT PER SERVING: 3.1 grams of carb, 6.5 grams of protein.
SERVING SIZE: one roll (of 12). AMOUNT PER SERVING: 4.2 grams of carb, 8.6 grams of protein.

	CHO (g)	PRO (g)
¾ cup cold water plus 2 tablespoons (this is important)	0	0
6 tablespoons butter (¾ stick)	0	0
¾ cup vital wheat gluten flour (see *Note*)	16.8	78.0
⅓ cup *unbleached*, all-purpose wheat (white) flour	30.7	4.0
trace of salt (two light shakes or to taste)	0	0
3 eggs*	1.8	18.0
1 egg white	0.3	3.5
Total	*49.6*	*103.5*

* If possible, weigh the eggs for this recipe. They should weigh between 62.0 grams and 64.0 grams (2.2 to 2.3 ounces). You can find these eggs among large and extra large eggs. If you have no scale, pick the smallest of the eggs in the carton.

Preheat oven to 425°F. Have ready one large, nonstick, heavy-gauge metal cookie sheet.

Put the water and the butter in a heavy 2-quart saucepan, preferably with a rounded bottom, over medium heat. Occasionally stir the mixture while you wait for the butter to melt.

Meanwhile, thoroughly combine the two flours, and a pinch of salt in a medium mixing bowl.

As soon as the butter has melted and the mixture begins to simmer, add the dry mix all at once, and stir vigorously with a wooden spoon. Within just a few seconds, the dough will become smooth and leave the bottom and sides of the pan. Keep stirring until no flour shows. Cook for about 10 seconds longer and remove from heat.

Put the hot saucepan on a cold burner or other safe surface. Stir in the eggs, one at a time, mixing well after each addition. At first the dough will appear lumpy. When the whole eggs have been added, the dough will be smooth. It should be creamy and hold peaks with almost no settling. Work in the egg white. Now the dough will be just right; it will still hold its shape, but in softer peaks. It should form mounds that do not spread on the cookie sheet, but sink back and broaden out slightly. Occasionally, you may need to make a judgment call. Depending on the size of the eggs, the dough may be sufficiently soft even before you add the final egg white. In that case, omit the egg white or add it by the tablespoon. The right consistency makes the best rolls. Dough that is too stiff results in smaller rolls; dough that is too soft (i.e., spreads out wide on the cookie sheet) may result in flat rolls.

If you like, use your electric mixer to work in the eggs. Simply transfer the hot dough from the saucepan to the mixer bowl and beat in the eggs, one at a time. Do not overbeat because if you do, the rolls may develop large air pockets. Use a flat beater if you have one.

Put spoonfuls of dough on the cookie sheet, choosing the size you prefer. Use large teaspoons or even soup spoons to drop the dough. Place them fairly close together.

Bake the rolls for about 25 to 28 minutes or until they are golden brown and crusty on top. Promptly freeze rolls that you do not plan to use the day they are baked. Take them out of the bag to thaw at room temperature. You can also put the frozen rolls in the oven, set at 350°F (no need to preheat), and bake for 5 minutes. You can toast rolls (slice

Note: You can use vital wheat gluten flour from any health food store or supermarket to make rolls. However, the flours vary slightly from manufacturer to manufacturer and some flours may not allow your rolls to rise quite as high as they should (taste is not affected). For consistently good results, you may want to order your flour from the sources listed in "Mail-Order Sources." They have the best price we have been able to find—even after shipping.

in half), but you need a wide-slot toaster or toaster oven. The rolls toast rapidly, so use the lowest setting.

Save unused rolls in a dry place until rock hard. They will be used for Bread Crumbs I, page 25.

Variation: **Whole-Wheat Magic Rolls**

You can impart a slightly heartier flavor to the Magic Rolls and turn the white dinner rolls into whole-wheat rolls. The rolls will remain light. The stoneground whole-wheat flour adds only 1.3 teaspoons of flour to each roll (out of a total of 18 rolls). Substitute ½ cup of stone-ground whole-wheat flour for ⅓ cup all-purpose wheat (white) flour. Otherwise, follow directions precisely. You only gain 6.2 grams of carb for the batch; each whole-wheat roll, based on a count of 18, has 3.1 grams of carb. The protein change is insignificant.

Variation: **Low-Carb Danish Pastry**

This is a delicious treat for an extra 1.9 grams of carb for a Magic Roll (of any size). All you do is add a glaze to the rolls once they are baked. Follow the directions for Magic Rolls on page 22. While the rolls are baking, make ½ or ¼ of the Sugar Glaze recipe on page 275. (You can also make a larger amount of glaze and store it in the fridge for several days.) Apply the glaze thinly with a pastry brush to the tops of the hot rolls. It will set within minutes. The rolls freeze well even with the glaze. Thaw at room temperature or follow directions for heating in the oven.

Variation: **Raisin Rolls**

Follow the directions for Magic Rolls on page 22. Once all the eggs have been worked into the dough, stir in 1½ ounces of raisins. The raisin rolls will not rise as high, but they will taste terrific. Bake the rolls at 425°F to 450°F for about 15 to 18 minutes and check early. For total extravagance you can add the raisins to Low-Carb Danish Pastry, page 24. Combining glaze and raisins raises total carb per roll, based on the 18-count, to 5.8 grams. But are they good!

Variation: **Herbed Croutons I**

Store-bought croutons average 16.0 to 18.0 grams of carb per cup. Croutons made from Magic Rolls have 3.6 grams of carb per cup. Five small or four medium Magic Rolls make about 4 cups of crou-tons. You can leave them plain, but they taste especially good with the addition of herbs and spices. Cut the rolls in cubes. (If the rolls are frozen, thaw them slightly.) The cubes will shrink, so cut them about one-third larger than the size you would like them to be. Preheat a large, heavy skillet over medium heat. Add 3 tablespoons olive oil and 2 tablespoons butter to the skillet. As soon as the butter begins to foam—do not let it brown—stir in 2 teaspoons dried basil and 1 tablespoon dried parsley. Add the croutons and stir rapidly to make sure that all pieces get coated quickly with herbs and fats. Sprinkle an optional ¼ teaspoon garlic powder over the croutons along with a little salt. Continue to stir until the croutons take on a light golden color. The herbs and garlic add about 2.0 grams of carb, or 0.5 grams per cup. Cool croutons. Store extra croutons in refrigerator or freeze. Put frozen croutons in a 350°F preheated oven for 5 minutes to restore crunch. PREPARATION TIME: 15 minutes.

Variation: Herbed Croutons II   *(gluten-free)*

These croutons are made from waffles (Basic Waffles, page 53 in Chapter 3). Follow the recipe for making Herbed Croutons I on page 24). It takes about six 4-inch square waffles or two 7½-inch round waffles to make 4 cups of croutons. The carb count per cup is 3.6 grams, protein 10.4 grams. Add 0.5 grams of carb for herbs.

Variation: Bread Crumbs I

Use leftover dry Magic Rolls for making bread crumbs. One cup of commercial bread crumbs has 76.0 grams of carb. A cup of bread crumbs made from Magic Rolls has 10.8 grams of carb and 22.8 grams of protein. Making bread crumbs is a cinch with a food processor. The crumbs keep practically forever at room temperature; you can also store them in the fridge or freezer. Collect leftover rolls until you have a sizable batch. Drop them in a container or into a roasting pan and cover with a light kitchen towel. Never store them airtight. Cut the dry rolls in halves or quarters and toss them in the food processor using the metal blade. Fill the processor (whatever size) about three-fourths full. Pulse to get fine crumbs. You can also put the chunks in a plastic bag and pound them with a meat mallet or use a rolling pin. The crumbs are more heat sensitive than regular bread crumbs, so reduce your heat setting slightly when cooking with them. PREPARATION TIME: Depends on number of rolls. Takes only two minutes per batch.

Variation: Bread Crumbs II *(gluten free)*

These bread crumbs are made from waffles (Basic Waffles, page 53 in Chapter 3). Follow the recipe for making Bread Crumbs I on page 25. It takes about four 4-inch square waffles or two 7½-inch round waffles to make 2 cups of bread crumbs. One cup has 9.6 grams of carb and 36.6 grams of protein. PREPARATION TIME: Same as for Bread Crumbs I.

Variation: Best Garlic Bread

This garlic bread is quick to make. Follow the directions for making Magic Rolls on page 22. You can use rolls of any size. Use two rolls per serving (or more). Preheat oven to 300°F or 325°F. For two or three servings of garlic bread, mix ⅓ cup butter with 8 teaspoons crushed garlic or 4 teaspoons powdered garlic. (1 teaspoon crushed garlic has 1.0 gram of carb; 1 teaspoon garlic powder has 2.3 grams of carb.) Slice each roll in four or five pieces and spread the garlic butter on one side only. Set the slices on a nonstick, heavy-gauge metal cookie sheet, garlic side up. For easier cleanup, first put a sheet of aluminum foil on the cookie sheet. Sprinkle grated Parmesan cheese on top of the garlic bread slices, using about 1 ounce. Bake for 10 to 12 minutes or until the slices have turned a golden color; the underside of the slices will also turn golden. Garlic and cheese add 9.0 grams of carb and 9.0 grams of protein. A single serving (based on two 3½-inch rolls) has 11.1 grams of carb and 18.5 grams of protein.

Cinnamon Walnut Power Muffins

This is a tasty, high-protein, anytime snack that will stick with you. The muffins are fiber-rich (2.5 grams per muffin). These large (2.5 ounces) muffins each have 5.5 grams of carb and 10.7 grams of protein.

PREPARATION TIME: 15 to 20 minutes. BAKING TIME: 20 to 25 minutes.
SERVING SIZE: one muffin. AMOUNT PER SERVING: 5.8 grams of carb, 10.6 grams of protein. NUMBER OF SERVINGS: 12.

		CHO (g)	PRO (g)
12	ounces cream cheese, soft	9.6	25.2
5	eggs	3.0	30.0
15	packets Splenda sugar substitute	15.0	0
2	teaspoons vanilla	1.0	0
1½	cups whole almond meal	18.0	36.0
1	cup unprocessed wheat bran	12.0	8.0
1	teaspoon baking powder	1.2	0
2	teaspoons ground cinnamon	1.4	0
1	cup chopped walnuts	8.0	27.6
	Total	*69.2*	*126.8*

Preheat oven to 325°F. Lightly grease a 12-cup muffin pan (heavy-gauge metal is best). You can also use muffin liners.

Put cream cheese and two eggs in the bowl of an electric mixer. Beat with a flat beater until smooth and fluffy. Add the other eggs, one at a time, beating briefly after each. On slow speed, stir in the rest of the ingredients except the walnuts. When mixture is well blended, stir in the walnuts.

Fill the muffin pans almost to the top. (The muffins will rise only slightly.) Bake muffins for about 20 to 25 minutes or until golden brown. These muffins freeze well. Thaw at room temperature.

Variation: Cranberry Power Muffins

Follow the Cinnamon Walnut Power Muffin recipe (above), but omit cinnamon and walnuts. Add 1 cup whole or coarsely chopped (fresh or frozen) cranberries to the batter. Fold berries in last. A cranberry muffin has 4.8 grams of carb and 8.5 grams of protein.

Variation: Blueberry Power Muffins

Follow the Cinnamon Walnut Power Muffin recipe (above), but omit cinnamon and walnuts. Add 1 cup whole blueberries (fresh or frozen) and 2 teaspoons grated lemon peel. A blueberry muffin has 5.6 grams of carb and 8.5 grams of protein.

Elegant Biscuits

Quick to make and delicious, each biscuit has 5.1 grams of carb. The biscuits freeze well and they are great toasted. If you like biscuits sweet, add 5 packets of Splenda sugar and adjust carb count.

PREPARATION TIME: 10 minutes. BAKING TIME: 11 to 15 minutes.
SERVING SIZE: one biscuit. AMOUNT PER SERVING: 5.1 grams of carb, 10.9 grams of protein. NUMBER OF SERVINGS: 10.

		CHO (g)	PRO (g)
⅓	cup vital wheat gluten flour	7.5	34.7
¼	cup unbleached, all-purpose wheat (white) flour	23.0	3.0
¼	cup soy protein powder	0	16.0
¼	cup whey protein powder	3.0	20.0
1	cup whole almond meal	12.0	24.0
1	teaspoon baking powder	1.2	0
1½	ounces butter, soft	0	0
1	egg	0.6	6.0
6	tablespoons light cream	2.4	1.8
2	tablespoons whole almond meal	1.5	3.0
	Total	*51.2*	*108.5*

Preheat oven to 300°F or 325°F. Have ready one large, nonstick, heavy-gauge metal cookie sheet.

Put the first six ingredients in a medium mixing bowl and mix well. Cut the butter into the dry mix in small chunks. Disperse the butter evenly with a pastry cutter or use your fingertips to get a crumbly mix (it takes a few seconds). In a small bowl stir together the egg and cream. Add to the dry mix. Stir lightly with a fork just to moisten. Continue by hand. Mix only until the dough *barely sticks together.* This is important. (Too much kneading results in dry and less flaky biscuits.) The dough should be soft.

Sprinkle 1 tablespoon of ground almonds on a cutting board or the countertop. Put the biscuit dough in a single slab on top of the nuts. Sprinkle another tablespoon of ground almonds on top of the dough. Pat dough down to about ¾-inch thickness. Cut 10 biscuits with a 2-inch biscuit cutter. You can also shape the biscuits by hand. Use a spatula to lift the biscuits onto the cookie sheet. Bake for about 11 to 15 minutes or until light golden.

Black Soybean Bread   *(gluten-free)*

This unusual and tasty bread is easy to make and is gluten-free. It is best baked in mini loaf pans (3 × 6 inches or similar). Use three pans for this recipe. Black soybeans are low in carbs and rich in fiber and protein. You can freeze this bread, too. One loaf has 11.7 grams of carb and 47.3 grams of protein. Try the bread toasted.

PREPARATION TIME: 20 minutes. BAKING TIME: 30 to 40 minutes.
SERVING SIZE: one slice. AMOUNT PER SERVING: 1.2 grams of carb, 4.8 grams of protein. NUMBER OF SERVINGS: 30.

		CHO (g)	PRO (g)
8	ounces cream cheese, soft	6.4	16.8
5	eggs	3.0	30.0
1	cup rinsed, lightly mashed organic black soybeans, drained	6.4	13.8
¼	cup whey protein powder	3.0	20.0
½	cup soy protein powder	0	32.0
1	teaspoon baking powder	1.2	0
	pinch of salt	0	0
1¼	cups whole almond meal	15.0	30.0
	Total	*35.0*	*142.6*

Preheat oven to 300°F or 325°F. Lightly butter three mini loaf pans (use nonstick pans made of heavy-gauge metal). For easy cleanup and removal, cut strips of waxed paper to fit in the bottom of the pans and allow them to hang over the edge by an inch or two.

Put cream cheese and two eggs in the bowl of an electric mixer and beat with a flat beater until smooth and fluffy. Add the remaining eggs, one at a time, beating briefly after each addition. Add the remaining ingredients and blend at low speed or by hand.

Spoon the batter into the pans and bake the bread for about 30 to 40 minutes or until done. Cool before slicing. Keep refrigerated (keeps for about 3 to 4 days). Freeze bread that isn't going to be used soon.

Super Banana Bread

Here is a yummy banana bread that has a rich banana flavor and is still fairly low-carb. It is wonderful for breakfast, too. Bake the bread in mini loaf pans (3 × 6 inches, or so) for best results. A slice of banana bread that weighs about 1.0 ounce has 4.5 grams of carb and 3.7 grams of protein. A commercial or homemade slice of banana bread of the same weight has about 16.0 grams of carb.

PREPARATION TIME: 30 minutes. BAKING TIME: 45 to 55 minutes.
SERVING SIZE: one ½-inch thick slice. AMOUNT PER SERVING: 4.4 grams of carb, 3.7 grams of protein. NUMBER OF SERVINGS: 30.

		CHO (g)	PRO (g)
12	ounces cream cheese, soft	9.6	25.2
5	eggs	3.0	30.0
1	cup mashed bananas (about 3 medium-size bananas)	54.0	2.7
¼	cup soy protein powder	0	16.0
⅓	cup stoneground whole-wheat flour	24.1	5.3
1	teaspoon baking powder	1.2	0
16	packets Splenda sugar substitute	16.0	0
2	teaspoons vanilla extract	1.0	0
2	teaspoons grated lemon peel (optional)	0.2	0
1	cup unprocessed wheat bran	12.0	8.0
1	cup whole almond meal	12.0	24.0
	Total	*132.0*	*108.9*

Preheat oven to 325°F. Lightly butter three miniloaf pans (use non-stick pans made of heavy-gauge metal). Optional: For easy cleanup and removal, cut strips of waxed paper to fit in the bottoms of the pans and allow them to hang over the edge by an inch or two.

Put cream cheese and two eggs in the bowl of an electric mixer and beat with a flat beater until smooth, thick, and fluffy. Be sure to eliminate all cream cheese lumps. Add the remaining eggs, one at a time, beating briefly after each addition. Add the next seven ingredients and beat at slow speed. Add the wheat bran and nuts, blending at low speed.

Spoon the batter into the pans and bake the banana bread for about 45 to 55 minutes or until done. Cool before slicing. Keep refrigerated (keeps for about 3 to 4 days). Freeze bread that isn't going to be used soon.

Variation: Lower-Carb Banana Bread

Omit stoneground whole-wheat flour. Increase the soy protein powder to ½ cup. It will reduce a slice of bread to 3.6 grams of carb. Protein for the slice is 4.1 grams.

Cranberry Bread

A great way to start the day, or eat this bread as an anytime snack. If you like the tart flavor of cranberries, you will love it. A slice of cranberry bread has 3.2 grams of carb and 3.9 grams of protein.

PREPARATION TIME: 20 minutes. BAKING TIME: 30 to 40 minutes.
SERVING SIZE: one slice. AMOUNT PER SERVING: 3.3 grams of carb, 3.9 grams of protein. NUMBER OF SERVINGS: 30.

		CHO (g)	PRO (g)
12	ounces cream cheese, soft	9.6	25.2
5	eggs	3.0	30.0
¼	cup vital wheat gluten flour	5.6	26.0
¼	cup unbleached, all-purpose wheat (white) flour	23.0	3.0
1	teaspoon baking powder	1.2	0
20	packets Splenda sugar substitute	20.0	0
1	cup unprocessed wheat bran	12.0	8.0
1	cup whole almond meal	12.0	24.0
1½	cups fresh or frozen cranberries, crushed lightly	12.0	0.6
	Total	*98.4*	*116.8*

Preheat oven to 300°F or 325°F. Lightly butter three miniloaf pans (use nonstick pans made of heavy-gauge metal). Optional: For easy cleanup and removal, cut strips of waxed paper to fit in the bottoms of the pans and allow them to hang over the edge by an inch or two.

Put cream cheese and two eggs in the bowl of an electric mixer and beat with a flat beater until smooth, thick, and fluffy. Add the remaining eggs, one at a time, beating briefly after each addition. Add the remaining ingredients except for the cranberries. Mix together at low speed. Then fold in the cranberries.

Spoon the batter into the pans and bake the cranberry bread for about 40 to 50 minutes or until done. Cool before slicing. Keep refrigerated (keeps for about 3 to 4 days). Freeze bread that isn't going to be used soon.

Variation: Whole-Wheat-Flour Cranberry Bread

Substitute ⅓ cup stoneground whole-wheat flour for ¼ cup wheat (white) flour. There is a negligible gain in total carb of 1.1 grams.

Butter Gems

Rich and flaky with a delicious buttery taste, these crackers are wonderful for just about any purpose including as plain munchies. One cracker has a mere 0.6 grams of carb.

PREPARATION TIME: 30 minutes. BAKING TIME: 45 minutes.
SERVING SIZE: one cracker. AMOUNT PER SERVING: 0.6 grams of carb, 0.8 grams of protein. NUMBER OF SERVINGS: 90 to 95.

		CHO (g)	PRO (g)
8	tablespoons butter (1 stick), soft	0	0
4	egg yolks	1.2	11.2
⅓	cup unbleached all-purpose wheat (white) flour	30.7	4.0
⅓	cup vital wheat gluten flour	7.5	34.8
	salt to taste		
	freshly ground black pepper to taste		
1	teaspoon baking powder	1.2	0
1	cup whole almond meal	12.0	24.0
	Total	*52.6*	*74.0*

Once prepared, the dough will need to be refrigerated, so preheat oven to 300°F or 325°F shortly before taking dough from fridge. Use two large, nonstick, heavy-gauge metal cookie sheets.

Combine butter and two egg yolks in the bowl of an electric mixer and beat with a flat beater until thick and creamy. Add the remaining yolks and beat some more. Add all the other ingredients, stirring in at low speed or by hand. Refrigerate dough for about 30 minutes or longer, until the dough firms up and can be handled without sticking.

Form balls the size of grapes and put them on a cookie sheet. Allow room for some expansion. Flatten each cracker slightly with your fingertips.

Bake the crackers for 9 to 11 minutes, one cookie sheet at a time. The crackers should be barely golden with a slightly darker edge (avoid having the edges turn too dark). These crackers are great keepers (even at room temperature). They freeze well, too.

LOW-CARB YEAST BREADS

The recipes in this book make the bread-baking process as close to being automatic as you can get without actually using a bread machine. Use your electric mixer if it has a dough hook or your food processor if it has an 11-cup capacity. Even hand-kneading takes only 5 minutes. You can have bread rising in the oven within 15 minutes. Once it's in there, all you do is give it time to grow; then you just bake away. You can make more than one type of bread (rolls, too); the process is always the same. The total amount of bread varies slightly from recipe to recipe. Some recipes yield a little less than 2 pounds; others a bit more. All recipes allow you to make two large or four small loaves.

The bread carb counts in this book range from 2.3 grams per ounce to 5.7 grams. Commercial bread slices have between 12.0 and 14.0 grams of carb per ounce. You may be surprised by how great these low-carb breads taste. That even goes for the incredible Almost No-Carb Bread (page 37). You'd never believe it has a mere 2.3 grams of carb in a 1-ounce slice. It is so delicious that you may be content to have it as your daily bread.

Best Whole-Wheat Bread

You can bake four small loaves or two large loaves. You can also shape the loaves any way you like without using a pan. Smaller loaves may help with carb control. Freeze loaves that you don't use right away. Two standard loaves made from this recipe weigh about 15 to 16 ounces each.

PREPARATION TIME: 15 to 20 minutes. BAKING TIME: 30 to 45 minutes (depending on size of loaves).

SERVING SIZE: one slice. AMOUNT PER SERVING: 3.7 grams of carb, 6.3 grams of protein. NUMBER OF SERVINGS: 29. Total yield: 30 to 32 ounces (2 large or 4 small loaves).

		CHO (g)	PRO (g)
¾	cup hot water	0	0
1	cup cold water	0	0
2	tablespoons olive oil	0	0
1	package rapid-rise yeast	1.2	0
1¼	cups whole almond meal	15.0	30.0
1¼	cups unprocessed wheat bran, toasted*	15.0	10.0
1⅓	cups vital wheat gluten flour	30.0	138.7
⅔	cup stoneground whole-wheat flour	48.3	10.9
	salt to taste (about ¾ teaspoon)		
	olive oil for kneading, as needed		
	Total	*109.5*	*189.6*

Preheat oven to 200°F when you begin making the bread. Turn oven off when you begin shaping the bread. Use butter or coconut oil to grease the nonstick, heavy-gauge metal bread pans that you intend to use or the cookie sheet if making free forms.

Combine the hot and cold water in the bowl of the electric mixer, food processor, or in a large mixing bowl. Add the oil. Stir in the yeast. Yeast will activate without adding sugar; give it about 5 minutes.

Meanwhile, put the dry ingredients in a medium mixing bowl and stir together. After 5 minutes, add the dry mixture to the liquid. Set the mixer on the lowest setting to knead the dough for 5 minutes. Pulse for about 1 minute if using a food processor. If the dry mixture is not fully absorbed (some of it remains visible at the bottom of the mixing bowl), add a tablespoon of warm water to the dough. If the dough is too loose, in which case it won't turn into a ball or at least hang together, add a tablespoon of soy protein powder. To make the dough

---

* You can toast wheat bran 3 or 4 cups at a time in a large, shallow baking pan for 25 to 30 minutes at 300°F. Do not let the bran get very dark. You can also buy Kretschmer's Toasted Wheat Bran; it is ready to go.

manually, stir the dry ingredients with a fork until the moisture is almost absorbed. Take over by hand and knead the dough for 5 or 6 minutes (no need to do more). The dough will start out rather squishy (not sticky) but will stiffen as you proceed. Periodically, pour a few drops of oil in the palms of your hands or over the dough; it will help keep the dough smooth and elastic.

Divide the dough in two or four equal portions. Shape into loaves. The dough should not be sticky but you can dust your palms with a bit of soy protein powder while shaping the loaves or use a bit of olive oil on your palms, if you like. Put loaves in the baking pans of your choice or free-form them. Before you put the loaves in the prewarmed oven, open the oven for about 30 seconds (the oven temperature should feel just a touch warm to your hand, not hot). (Even if you forgot to turn the oven off earlier, the open door will make the temperature plummet promptly.) Let the loaves rise for about 60 to 75 minutes (they will almost triple in bulk). After the breads have risen, set oven temperature to 350°F (do not remove bread). Bake the loaves for 30 minutes for small loaves or until done and for 40 to 45 minutes for large loaves. The crust should be crisp, light brown, and feel hollow to the touch. Wait for the bread to cool completely before slicing.

Freeze extra loaves. Thaw loaves at room temperature. They will be perfect. Avoid using a microwave for thawing or warming. This bread also tastes simply delicious toasted.

Variation: **Pumpernickel Bread**

This is a very dark, dense bread with an incredibly delicious flavor. No one will believe that it is low-carb. Pine nuts add to the flavor and interesting texture; cocoa powder adds to the color. Follow the recipe for Best Whole-Wheat Bread and for Gourmet Rye Bread, but increase hot water to 1 cup. Reduce almond meal to 1 cup; increase crude wheat bran to 1¾ cups; increase vital wheat gluten flour to 1½ cups. Add ¼ cup unsweetened cocoa. Add pine nuts to taste—about ¼ cup. Total carbs for the bread are 122.9 grams; total protein is 227.7 grams. Total weight is 36.0 ounces. A 1-ounce slice of bread has 3.5 grams of carb and 6.7 grams of protein.

Variation: **Raisin Wheat Bread**

Follow the directions for Best Whole-Wheat Bread on page 34, but add ½ cup washed and drained raisins to the dough along with the dry flour mix. Total carbs for this recipe increase to 165.6 grams. One slice of bread has 5.0 grams of carb and the protein gain is insignificant. The total yield is 33 slices.

Variation: Gourmet Rye Bread

This is a delicious bread with a wonderful rye flavor. Simply follow the directions for making Best Whole-Wheat Bread (page 34) and substitute ¾ cup dark rye flour for the stoneground whole-wheat flour. The change in carbs and protein is negligible.

Variation: Rye Bread with Caraway

Caraway seeds make a great addition to this bread and give it a change of flavor. Add 1 or 2 tablespoons of caraway to the dry mix when you prepare the bread. One tablespoon of caraway seeds has 1.6 grams of carb.

Variation: Hearty Country Rolls

Follow the directions for making Best Whole-Wheat Bread dough on page 34. Use it or any of the variations for making rolls.

Divide the dough into four equal portions, then divide each of these into five sections. Form rolls and set them on a greased, non-stick, heavy-gauge metal cookie sheet or jelly roll pan. Allow rolls to rise in the oven just as you would bread (same amount of time). Reduce baking time to about 18 to 22 minutes or until rolls are done. Freeze excess rolls promptly. Thaw at room temperature. The carb count per roll is based on the recipe you choose. Divide total carbs and protein by 20.

Variation: Sourdough Rye Bread

Follow the directions for making Gourmet Rye Bread (above), but the night before you plan to bake Sourdough Rye Bread, combine ½ cup cold water, ½ cup boiling water, ½ cup sour cream, 1 table-spoon olive oil, and 1 package dry yeast (not rapid-rise) in a large mixing bowl (this starter mix will more than double in bulk overnight). Add ¾ cup dark rye flour and beat well. Cover the bowl tightly and keep at room temperature overnight. Preheat oven for 15 minutes to 200°F and turn off. In a medium mixing bowl, combine almond meal, vital wheat gluten flour, toasted wheat bran, and salt. Add ¼ cup hot water to the starter bowl; stir down. If you plan to use the electric mixer, prepare the starter directly in the mixer bowl. Add the dry ingredients. Continue to follow the directions for making Gourmet Rye Bread. The total amount of bread and the carb and protein counts remain essentially the same as those for Whole-Wheat Bread (total carbs: 107.7 grams, protein: 205.8 grams).

Almost No-Carb Bread

Follow the directions for making Best Whole-Wheat Bread (page 34) except for the change in ingredients as follows. Blanched almond flour creates a light texture. For occasional variety, try using it instead of whole almond meal.

SERVING SIZE: one slice. AMOUNT PER SERVING: 2.7 grams of carb, 8.1 grams of protein. NUMBER OF SERVINGS: 33. TOTAL YIELD: 33 to 34 ounces (2 large or 4 small loaves).

		CHO (g)	PRO (g)
1¼	cups cold water	0	0
1	cup hot water	0	0
2	tablespoons olive oil	0	0
1	package rapid-rise yeast	1.2	0
1¼	cups whole almond meal	15.0	30.0
1¾	cups unprocessed wheat bran, toasted	21.0	14.0
1½	cups vital wheat gluten flour	33.6	156.0
1	cup soy protein powder	0	64.4
¼	cup stoneground whole-wheat flour	18.1	4.0
	salt to taste (about ¾ teaspoon)	0	0
	olive oil for kneading, as needed	0	0
	Total	*88.9*	*268.4*

Can't-Believe Cinnamon Buns

This delicious cinnamon bun has 6.3 grams of carb if baked in a 12-cup muffin pan. Commercial cinnamon buns of approximately the same weight—Pepperidge Farm Cinnamon Rolls, for example—have 23.0 grams of carb. You can also make smaller buns and more of them, dropping the carb count. For example, 18 buns would have 4.2 grams of carb each.

PREPARATION TIME: 25 minutes. BAKING TIME: 15 to 20 minutes.

SERVING SIZE: one bun. AMOUNT PER SERVING: 6.3 grams of carb, 8.3 grams of protein. NUMBER OF SERVINGS: 12 or more.

		CHO (g)	PRO (g)
½	cup hot water	0	0
3	tablespoons butter, soft	0	0
3	tablespoons cold water	0	0
2	teaspoons vanilla extract	1.0	0
5	packets Splenda sugar substitute	5.0	0
1	package rapid-rise yeast	1.2	0
⅓	cup unbleached, all-purpose wheat (white) flour	30.7	4.0
¼	cup vital wheat gluten flour	5.6	26.0
1¼	cups whole almond meal	15.0	30.0
½	cup soy protein powder	0	32.0
	pinch of salt	0	0
2	tablespoons soy protein powder for rolling dough	0	8.0
FILLING			
1	tablespoon ground cinnamon	2.1	0
15	packets Splenda sugar substitute	15.0	0
1	tablespoon butter, soft	0	0
	Total	*75.6*	*100.0*

Preheat oven to 200°F for 15 minutes and turn off. Lightly butter a 12-cup muffin pan (heavy-gauge metal is best) or use muffin liners. If you want to make more than 12 buns—they will be smaller—use a nonstick, heavy-gauge metal cookie sheet.

Mix cinnamon and Splenda sugar substitute for the filling.* Have ready.

Put the hot water in the bowl of your electric mixer or processor. You can use a 7-cup processor or a medium mixing bowl if you do this by hand. Add the butter and stir until dissolved. Add cold water, vanilla extract, Splenda sugar substitute, and yeast. Stir, then wait 5 minutes.

Meanwhile, combine the remaining ingredients except for the last two tablespoons of soy protein powder in a mixing bowl and stir. Add to the liquid. Knead the dough in the mixer for about 5 minutes or about 1 minute in the processor. (If you do not have a dough hook, you can use a flat beater. This is a relatively small amount of dough.) If you do it manually, stir mixture with a fork until combined and take over by hand. Knead dough for 5 minutes. (If needed, rub a bit of either soy protein powder or olive oil on your palms.)

Put the dough on a large cutting board. Put a kitchen towel under the board so that it won't move around. Spread out 2 teaspoons of soy protein powder (add more if needed; you should not need much). Shape the dough roughly into a rectangle with your hands before applying the rolling pin. Roll out a 12- by 16-inch sheet. If the edges are too ragged, cut off pieces of dough here and there and attach where needed. Press down and continue to roll out. Make the sheet larger for more buns.

Brush sheet with 1 tablespoon soft butter. Sprinkle evenly with the cinnamon-sugar mix. Begin rolling from one end. Form a tight roll. Cut it in two sections. Elongate each section a little (by squeezing); cut each in six equal portions and set them in the muffin pan. If you want to make more buns, cut the roll of dough in three pieces and elongate each by squeezing. Cut in slices and put them on a cookie sheet. Allow to rise for about 35 to 40 minutes in the prewarmed oven. To bake, set temperature to 325°F. Bake for 15 to 20 minutes or until done. Cool. These rolls freeze well. Thaw at room temperature.

Variation: Nutty Cinnamon Buns

Add ¾ cup chopped pecans or walnuts. Sprinkle them evenly over the surface of the dough after you have applied butter, cinnamon, and sugar. This adds 0.5 grams of carb per cinnamon bun (if you make 12) and 1.7 grams of protein, if you use walnuts. Pecans add 0.8 grams of protein.

Note: Adjust sweetener as desired for the filling. One packet of Splenda has 1.0 gram of carb. If you prefer to use real sugar (sucrose), omit the Splenda. Do not add sugar to the dough. Mix 4 tablespoons sugar (48.0 grams of carb) with the cinnamon. There is a net gain of 28 grams of carb. One cinnamon bun (of 12) will have 8.6 grams of carb.

3

LOW-CARB COMFORT FOOD BREAKFASTS, BRUNCHES, AND LIGHT MEALS

If you're new to the low-carb life, it probably seems exciting and even exotic to treat yourself to a couple of eggs with a side of bacon, sausage, or ham—all foods forbidden on low-fat regimes. It may, at first, seem too good to be true that you can eat steak and eggs or cheese omelets day after day and stick to your diet. But once you become a veteran of low-carb eating, you may find yourself staring at your plate of fried eggs, singing the low-carb breakfast blues as you wistfully long for the waffles, pancakes, blintzes, and French toast of yore.

Well, heat up the griddle and pull out the waffle iron. We're back in business with breakfast ideas that include French toast, multiple kinds of waffles, crepes, pancakes, and blintzes that are soft on carbs and strong on protein. Finally, you can feel good about a breakfast of pancakes, sausage, and fruit. If strawberry waffles ring your chimes, dig in. They're delicious, nutritious, and totally guilt-free.

You'll find the recipes in this breakfast section unbelievably easy. In no time at all, you'll whip up a batch of pancakes that will make a lazy Sunday morning feel like the good old days. And the great thing is, you won't jeopardize your low-carb commitment to leanness and good health. Get cooking!

Melt-in-Your-Mouth Pancakes   *(gluten-free)*

They really do melt in your mouth and are about as easy to make as stuff you pour from a container. Serve them with butter and carb-free or low-carb syrups, fresh fruit, Uncooked Blueberry Sauce (page 300), or Rhubarb Sauce (page 299). If all you want to eat is pancakes, the recipe serves one. Combined with sausage, ham, or something else, this is a serving for two.

PREPARATION TIME: 5 minutes. COOKING TIME: 3 to 4 minutes.
SERVING SIZE: three to four 3-inch pancakes. AMOUNT PER SERVING: 2.6 grams of carb, 15.1 grams of protein. NUMBER OF SERVINGS: 1 to 2.

	CHO (g)	PRO (g)
2 eggs	1.2	12.0
¼ cup soy protein powder	0	16.0
⅓ cup sour cream	2.7	2.1
1 teaspoon baking powder	1.2	0
2 tablespoons olive oil	0	0
Total	*5.1*	*30.1*

Preheat a heavy, nonstick, large griddle over medium to medium-low heat.

Combine ingredients in a small mixing bowl. Beat vigorously with a fork or wire whisk until the batter is well mixed and smooth.

Spoon batter onto the hot ungreased griddle (it is hot enough when a drop of water splashed on it bounces around). Allow for expansion of pancakes. (Note the batter is a bit on the thin side; that's okay.) Watch for bubbles and a hint of dryness on top before turning. The pancakes tend to darken more quickly than other pancakes you may be used to, so check early.

Variation: Richer Whey Pancakes

If you prefer, you can omit the soy protein powder and replace it with ⅓ cup whey protein powder. There is a net gain of 4.0 grams of carb and 6.7 grams of protein. A single serving of pancakes has 9.1 grams of carb and 37.7 grams of protein.

Variation: Cottage Cheese Pancakes

Adding cottage cheese directly to the pancake batter gives pancakes a slightly different, pleasant flavor. The carb count per single serving goes to 7.1 grams and protein goes to 37.1 grams. Add ¼ cup (4% butterfat) cottage cheese to the batter (if the cottage cheese is not dry, drain it thoroughly by pressing down on it).

Low-Carb Crepes

(gluten-free)

Crepes can be served individually as they come from the griddle or made ahead and kept warm in the oven or quickly reheated in the microwave. Crepes are a quick and acceptable substitute for pasta. They are featured in various desserts and as savory dishes. Because they are so easy to make, they are handy for wrap-arounds. Although not like tortillas, you can wrap your favorite tortilla fillings in them. You can be extremely creative with crepes without expending much effort. One crepe has 1.0 grams of carb and 5.9 grams of protein. Suggested breakfast crepe fillings begin on page 47. Although the directions for making crepes are quite long, it is simply to ensure that you do it right the first time. This recipe is easy to multiply.

PREPARATION TIME: 5 minutes. COOKING TIME: 90 seconds or less per crepe. SERVING SIZE: three 8-inch crepes. AMOUNT PER SERVING: 3.5 grams of carb, 20.7 grams of protein. NUMBER OF SERVINGS: 2. TOTAL YIELD: 7 crepes. (Carb and protein counts for fillings must be added separately.)

	CHO (g)	PRO (g)
4 eggs (or 1 cup egg substitute)	2.4	24.0
2 egg whites	0.6	7.0
⅓ cup sour cream	2.7	2.1
2 tablespoons soy protein powder	0	8.0
½ teaspoon baking powder	1.2	0
1 tablespoon water	0	0
butter for cooking, as needed	0	0
Total	*6.9*	*41.1*

Put all ingredients except the butter in a food processor or blender. Process briefly (only for about 10 to 12 seconds). Overbeating makes the batter foamy. You can also beat the batter by hand in a small mixing bowl; use a wire whisk. When you do this, tiny (sour cream) lumps usually persist. Ignore them; they disappear in cooking.

Preheat a nonstick 10-inch griddle (most 10-inch griddles make about 8½-inch or slightly larger crepes) over low to medium-low heat.

Melt a little butter on the griddle. Keep heat low enough so that the butter does not brown right away. When the butter foams, lift the pan with one hand and pour the batter in it with the other. Tilt the pan as you do this and swirl the batter around so that it coats the bottom

Note: Preheat oven to 200°F if you want to make the crepes ahead and keep them warm in the oven until all are cooked.

evenly and thinly. It takes about 3 tablespoons of batter to coat a 10-inch griddle. Experience will quickly guide you.

Cook the crepe until the outer edge shows a bit of dryness and a hint of color. Turn the crepe, using a 3-inch spatula. Crepes will always turn out—the difference is chiefly between good and superb. Cook them as briefly as possible. It's better to turn a crepe too soon— occasionally one may break—rather than wait too long. A broken crepe tastes just as good. Once turned, heat the crepe for only a few seconds. This side merely needs drying (it stays a light color).

It is simple to fill a crepe. Most commonly, a strip of filling is placed down the middle; the crepe is rolled like a jelly roll or you can fold the two side flaps over the center. You can also distribute the filling over most of the crepe and roll it like a jelly roll. You can spread the filling over half the crepe and fold over the other half, creating a pocket as if doing an omelet. You can also stack the crepes on top of one another, with fillings placed in between, and cut in wedges.

Variation: Whey Crepes

You can substitute about 3 tablespoons whey protein powder for soy protein powder. The total increase in carbs is only 2.3 grams, or a mere 0.3 grams per crepe. There is an insignificant increase in protein.

Note: Although crepes are traditionally thin, you can for the fun of it make them fairly thick and more like a pancake. Instead of rolling them up, put a filling on top or simply sprinkle with a little sugar or sugar substitute.

SWEET FILLINGS FOR CREPES

Generally, you need very little filling for great results, especially with bright, strong flavors from fruit. One large sliced strawberry, or eight raspberries, for example, are all you may need and perhaps add a sprinkling of Splenda sugar substitute. Often you can keep the filling per crepe under 1.0 gram of carb, or under 2.0 grams if you use additional sweetener. Fresh fruits give you the best (sweet) carb bargain. For your convenience, some carb grams are listed here for both fresh fruit and cooked fruits, followed by Cottage Cheese Crepes or Blintzes (page 48) and Banana Cream Crepe Filling (page 49).

FRESH FRUIT FILLINGS

Raspberries: 1 cup has 5.9 grams of carb; 10 berries have 0.9 grams of carb.

Strawberries: 1 cup (sliced) has 7.8 grams of carb; 1 medium-size strawberry has 0.6 grams of carb.

Boysenberries: 1 cup has 10.5 grams of carb.

Blueberries: 1 cup has 16.0 grams of carb.

Peaches: 1 cup (sliced) has 15.5 grams of carb.

Grapes: 1 cup, red or green, seedless (Thompson's) has 26.8 grams of carb; 1 grape has 0.8 grams of carb.

Cantaloupe: 1 cup (diced) has 11.8 grams of carb.

Honeydew: 1 cup (diced) has 14.6 grams of carb.

COOKED OR CANNED FRUIT FILLINGS

Rhubarb sauce (page 299): 2 tablespoons (unsweetened) have 0.6 grams of carb.

Cranberry sauce (page 299): 2 tablespoons (unsweetened) have 0.8 grams of carb.

Applesauce: 2 tablespoons (unsweetened) have 3.1 grams of carb.

Cottage Cheese Crepe Filling *(also called blintzes)*

PREPARATION TIME: 5 minutes. BAKING TIME: 15 minutes.
SERVING SIZE: about ⅓ cup, total yield. AMOUNT PER SERVING: 5.2 grams of
carb, 11.9 grams of protein. NUMBER OF SERVINGS: 2.

	CHO (g)	PRO (g)
¾ cup cottage cheese (4% butterfat, very dry)	6.0	21.0
1 egg yolk	0.3	2.8
1 teaspoon grated lemon peel	0.1	0
4 packets Splenda sugar substitute	4.0	0
Total	*10.4*	*23.8*

Preheat oven to 325°F. Line an 8- by 12-inch baking pan with aluminum foil.

Drain cottage cheese if necessary. Mix all of the ingredients together. Divide the filling evenly among four crepes (or as desired), placing the amounts as center strips on each. Roll the crepes like jelly rolls. Put them side by side in the baking pan and bake for about 15 minutes.

Banana Cream Crepe Filling

Prepare this filling before you make the crepes.

PREPARATION TIME: 5 minutes.
SERVING SIZE: ½ cup. AMOUNT PER SERVING: 9.1 grams of carb, 1.5 grams of
protein. NUMBER OF SERVINGS: 2.

		CHO (g)	PRO (g)
2	ounces mashed ripe banana	12.0	0.6
½	cup light or heavy cream	3.2	2.4
2	packets Splenda sugar substitute	2.0	0
2	teaspoons vanilla extract	1.0	0
	Total	*18.2*	*3.0*

Mash the banana. Beat the whipping cream until fairly stiff. Mix
with banana, Splenda sugar substitute, and vanilla extract. Divide the
filling among the centers of four crepes, roll up, and serve.

SAVORY FILLINGS FOR CREPES

These fillings are wonderful if you do not like sweet things for breakfast. All of them can be served at lunchtime as well or even as a light supper. Just combine with a hearty green salad.

Beef and Mushroom Crepe Filling

PREPARATION AND COOKING TIME: 15 minutes.
SERVING SIZE: ½ total yield. AMOUNT PER SERVING: 3.2 grams of carb, 15.5 grams of protein. NUMBER OF SERVINGS: 2.

	CHO (g)	PRO (g)
1 tablespoon olive oil or coconut oil	0	0
3 ounces lean ground beef	0	20.0
½ cup chopped scallions	2.4	0.9
4 ounces sliced mushrooms	4.0	2.0
salt to taste	0	0
freshly ground black pepper to taste	0	0
Total	*6.4*	*22.9*

Heat a small or medium skillet over medium heat. Add olive oil or coconut oil. Cook ground beef in hot oil until done. Set aside and keep warm. Add scallions to the skillet and cook for 1 minute. Add mushrooms and cook until just tender, about 4 to 5 minutes. Return meat to pan. Mix with onions and mushrooms; season to taste.

Put filling in the center of four crepes, roll up crepes, and serve.

Breakfast Sausage Crepe Filling

Use small sausages, about 20.0 grams each.

PREPARATION AND COOKING TIME: Follow package directions. Frozen sausages take about 7 to 8 minutes in a skillet or 5 minutes in a microwave. SERVING SIZE: about four sausages (20.0 grams each). AMOUNT PER SERVING: 3.0 grams of carb, 9.4 grams of protein. NUMBER OF SERVINGS: 2.

	CHO (g)	PRO (g)
8 small, fully cooked sausages	5.3	18.7
Total	*5.3*	*18.7*

Cook the sausages according to directions for the brand you use and compare carb and protein content. Slice the sausages in bite-size pieces and put two sausages inside each crepe. Roll up crepes and serve. This meal is excellent with a side of fresh, ripe peaches (but account for added carbs).

Veggie Cheese Crepe Filling

PREPARATION TIME: 10 minutes. COOKING TIME: 5 minutes. BAKING TIME: 15 to 20 minutes.

SERVING SIZE: ½ total yield. AMOUNT PER SERVING: 8.4 grams of carb, 16.8 grams of protein. NUMBER OF SERVINGS: 2.

	CHO (g)	PRO (g)
2 tablespoons olive oil or butter	0	0
¼ cup chopped onion	2.8	0
¾ cup chopped green bell peppers	3.5	0.6
¾ cup chopped red or orange bell peppers	3.5	0.6
salt to taste	0	0
freshly ground black pepper to taste	0	0
4 ounces shredded Swiss cheese	4.0	32.4
Total	*13.8*	*33.6*

Preheat oven to 325°F. Butter or oil an 8- by 12-inch baking pan or dish (or line with aluminum foil).

Heat a heavy skillet over medium heat. Add olive oil or butter. When the skillet is hot (do not brown butter), sauté onion for 1 or 2 minutes. Add peppers and sauté for about 2 to 3 minutes (keep peppers fairly crisp). Season with salt and pepper. Place fillings in center of four crepes (or as desired); sprinkle cheese over each filling. Roll the crepes like jelly rolls and place side by side in the baking dish. Bake for 15 to 20 minutes.

Low-Carb Waffles

Low-carb waffles are amazingly versatile. Most of these waffles are also gluten-free. A stale waffle can be made into gluten-free Bread Crumbs II (page 26) or turned into gluten-free Herbed Croutons II (page 25). Soak waffles in beaten egg and you get French Toast (page 57). You can choose from basic waffles, cheese waffles, and sourdough waffles. Dessert waffles are found in Chapter 9. Use low-carb or no-carb syrups (or pile on fruit or whipped cream or both). You can use the Fruit Fillings for Crepes on page 47. Try the Chocolate Hazelnut Spread (page 298) or Imitation Nutella. Waffles also make great underpinnings to many savory foods, including pizza.

The waffles tend to cook faster than regular waffles. Some are ready in 2 minutes, depending on your waffle maker. Always check early. It will not hurt to peek while steam is still coming out. Waffle makers vary in the size and depth of the waffles they produce. To get an accurate per-waffle carb and protein count, keep track of the number of waffles you get from a recipe. You only need to do this once. Divide your waffle output by the total carb and protein grams. All types of waffles can be frozen. Thaw before toasting.

Basic Waffles   *(gluten-free)*

PREPARATION TIME: 10 minutes. TOTAL BAKING TIME: about 15 minutes (depends on waffle maker).

SERVING SIZE: about two 4-inch square waffles or one 7½-inch round waffle (or equivalent). AMOUNT PER SERVING: 4.8 grams of carb, 18.3 grams of protein. NUMBER OF SERVINGS: 6 or 7.

		CHO (g)	PRO (g)
6	ounces cream cheese, soft	4.8	12.6
5	eggs*	3.0	30.0
¼	cup soy protein powder†	0	16.0
1	teaspoon baking powder	1.2	0
1¼	cup whole almond meal	15.0	30.0
¼	cup whey protein powder	3.0	20.0
¼	cup heavy cream	1.6	1.2
	Total	*28.6*	*109.8*

* For slightly lighter waffles, separate three of the five eggs. Add the yolks along with the whole eggs and beat the three egg whites. Fold in last.

† You can increase total whey protein powder to ½ cup and omit the soy protein powder. It adds 3.0 grams of carb to the total count.

In an electric mixer, food processor, or by hand, beat the cream cheese and two eggs until smooth, thick, and fluffy. Add the remaining three eggs, one at a time, beating briefly after each addition. Stir the soy protein powder, whey protein powder, baking powder, almond meal, whipping cream, and melted butter into the batter by hand or at slow mixer speed.

Spoon batter into the waffle iron. Bake until done (generally from 2 to 4 minutes). Always check early. The waffles are delicate, so remove them carefully. Do not pile them on top of one another or they may become soggy. You can freeze leftover waffles and heat them in a toaster (thaw first).

Variation: High-Fiber Waffles

These waffles have a delicious, hearty flavor. They are great as a base for savory toppings and for Personal Waffle Pizza (page 185), although they are not gluten-free. They are good with sweet toppings too. Follow the directions for making the Basic Waffles (page 53). Omit soy protein powder; reduce whole almond meal to ½ cup; add 1 cup unprocessed wheat bran, toasted or plain. Total yield is six or seven servings. A serving has 5.3 grams of carb and 14.6 grams of protein. The fiber provides 4.0 grams per serving.

Variation: Cheddar Cheese Waffles

Follow the directions for Basic Waffles (page 53), and add 4 ounces grated sharp cheddar cheese to the batter. Fold the cheese into the prepared batter and cook as directed. The cheese adds 1.6 grams of carb and 28.4 grams of protein to the recipe. A serving (based on 7) has 7.6 grams of carb and 19.7 grams of protein.

Note: If you plan to dry leftover waffles for crumbs or croutons, set them in a baking pan and keep them a bit separated for air circulation. Cover lightly with paper towels or kitchen towels.

Perfect Sourdough (Raised) Waffles

If you are not normally a waffle fan, these sourdough waffles are almost sure to make you one. They are crisp, delicate, with a slight yeasty flavor. You do not need a sourdough starter that you keep on hand in the fridge and nurture carefully. Instead you start the dough fresh each time you make these waffles. (It takes less than 10 minutes the night before to whip up the starter.) The batter keeps for about a week in the fridge—you can have another meal if you do not use all the batter at once. Freeze leftover waffles for future use. Heat in toaster (thaw first).

PREPARATION TIME: 10 minutes to make starter the night before. The following morning, 10 minutes. TOTAL COOKING TIME: 15 minutes (depends on waffle maker).

SERVING SIZE: two 4-inch square waffles or one 7-inch round waffle. AMOUNT PER SERVING: 4.5 grams of carb, 8.9 grams of protein. NUMBER OF SERVINGS: 10 or 11.

	CHO (g)	PRO (g)
⅓ cup boiling water	0	0
3 tablespoons butter	0	0
⅓ cup cold water	0	0
1 packet dry yeast	1.2	0
½ cup sour cream*	4.0	3.2
¼ cup stoneground whole-wheat flour†	18.1	4.0
¼ cup vital wheat gluten flour	5.6	26.0
4 eggs	2.4	24.0
¼ cup whey protein powder	6.0	20.0
1 teaspoon baking powder	1.2	0
½ cup whole almond meal	6.0	12.0
Total	*44.5*	*89.2*

The night before you plan to make the waffles, put the boiling water in a medium or large mixing bowl; add the butter and stir or beat until it is dissolved. Add the cold water. Add the yeast and stir. Wait 5 minutes. With a balloon whisk, beat in the sour cream, stoneground whole-wheat flour, and vital wheat gluten flour. Tightly cover the bowl. Let the starter sit at room temperature overnight.

---

* If it concerns you to have sour cream sit at room temperature overnight, leave out the sour cream at this point. You can add it in the morning. The early addition of the sour cream brings out a slightly more intense flavor. Note that the starter batter will be a little stiffer if it was prepared without the sour cream.

† You can use unbleached wheat (white) flour instead of stoneground whole-wheat flour. Just substitute one for the other. The white flour adds 4.9 grams of carb to the total carb count.

When you are ready to make waffles, preheat the waffle iron.

Beat the starter mixture until it is smooth (it will be almost double in bulk but will collapse). If you did not do it the night before, add the sour cream now. Beat the eggs into the mixture one at a time. Follow with the whey protein powder, baking powder, and whole almond meal. Beat until well mixed.

Spoon batter into the waffle iron. These waffles take perhaps a minute longer to bake than the other waffles in this cookbook. Still, the time is short. Remove waffles carefully. Do not pile them on top of one another or they may become soft.

Low-Carb French Toast

(gluten-free)

This French toast employs waffles instead of white or French bread and you will love it. You can use any waffles from this book. If you are using frozen waffles for making French toast, let them sit until all ice crystals have evaporated or stick them in the oven for a few minutes at 250°F.

PREPARATION TIME: 3 minutes with waffles on hand and thawed. COOKING TIME: 4 to 6 minutes.

SERVING SIZE: two 4-inch square waffles or one 7½-inch round waffle. AMOUNT PER SERVING: 6.2 grams of carb, 30.9 grams of protein. NUMBER OF SERVINGS: 1.

	CHO (g)	PRO (g)
1 7½-inch round waffle (or equivalent)	4.8	18.3
2 eggs	0.6	12.0
2 tablespoons light cream	0.8	0.6
1 tablespoon butter (or as desired)	0	0
Total	*6.2*	*30.9*

Lightly beat eggs and cream. Pour mixture in a pan that will hold the waffle. Turn the waffle two or three times to allow it to absorb the eggs. (All the egg mix will not be absorbed.)

Heat a large skillet over medium-low heat and melt butter in the skillet. When the butter foams (do not brown), add the waffle. Pour any egg not absorbed by the waffle over the top. Cook waffle slowly on one side until the egg is cooked. Turn and cook slowly on the other side. Serve immediately with a favorite low-carb syrup.

Crunchy Cereal

(gluten-free)

Here is a cereal that can help you out of the cereal blues. It delivers a nice crunch, a nice flavor—and few carbs. The basic ingredients are dried and chopped or lightly crushed waffles mixed with chopped nuts (7.0 grams of carb). One tablespoon of raisins will make a delicious addition. You can use any waffles as long as they are very dry. The recipe multiplies easily. Sprinkle with cinnamon or add some fresh fruit in season. Count all extra carbs. You can store the dry cereal for several weeks.

PREPARATION TIME: 5 minutes.

SERVING SIZE: 1¼ cups. AMOUNT PER SERVING: 9.0 grams of carb, 21.3 grams of protein. NUMBER OF SERVINGS: 1.

	CHO (g)	PRO (g)
2 4-inch square Basic Waffles (page 53) or equivalent	4.8	18.3
¼ cup chopped pecans	2.0	3.0
2 packets Splenda sugar substitute	2.0	0
¼ teaspoon cinnamon (optional)	0.2	0
Total	*9.0*	*21.3*

Crush the waffles very coarsely in a food processor, blender, or plastic bag. Use a rolling pin or meat mallet for the latter. Combine with the chopped pecans and serve in a bowl. Sprinkle Splenda and cinnamon on top. Serve with half and half cream diluted with water.

Note: One ounce of half and half has 1.3 grams of carb; 1 ounce of cream has 0.4 grams of carb. If you dilute the cream with a small amount of water to taste or even half and half, the carb cost will be quite low. Use sparingly because the cream is rich. If you use ½ cup regular or low-fat milk, you will gain an added 2.0 to 2.5 grams of carb.

Crouton Egg Bake

With a small amount of effort, you can have eggs cooked on a bed of toasted croutons and topped with cheese—a great leisurely breakfast or brunch. You can easily adjust this recipe for more or fewer people. If you don't have croutons ready, follow the directions in Chapter 2 for making Herbed Croutons I (page 24) or Herbed Croutons II (page 25).

PREPARATION TIME: 10 minutes. BAKING TIME: 15 minutes. (If croutons must be made, add 10 minutes to the preparation time.)

SERVING SIZE: 1 ramekin. AMOUNT PER SERVING: 2.6 grams of carb, 17.8 grams of protein. NUMBER OF SERVINGS: 4.

		CHO (g)	PRO (g)
1	cup herbed croutons	3.5	7.1
4	teaspoons freshly chopped parsley (or 1 teaspoon dried)	0	0
8	eggs	4.8	48.0
	salt to taste	0	0
	freshly ground black pepper to taste	0	0
4	ounces grated Swiss cheese (or other cheese of choice)	2.0	16.2
1	teaspoon butter (or as desired)	0	0
	Total	*10.3*	*71.3*

Preheat oven to 325°F. Lightly butter or oil four 4-inch ovenproof ramekins or bowls.

Put one-fourth of the croutons on the bottom of each ramekin. For each of 4 ramekins, break two eggs into a separate bowl and slide them on top of the croutons into each ramekin. Pierce yolks with a toothpick. Season eggs to taste with salt and freshly ground pepper. Sprinkle with cheese and parsley and dot with butter (optional). Bake until the eggs are set. Depending on how firm you want the eggs to be, this takes about 15 minutes or a little longer. Serve immediately.

Mustard-Baked Eggs

These mustard-baked eggs are extremely easy to prepare and can give a special flair to breakfast with nothing more than a touch of mustard and some cheese and cream. You'll want to make this dish often—and not necessarily just for breakfast.

PREPARATION TIME: 10 minutes. BAKING TIME: 15 minutes.
SERVING SIZE: 1 ramekin. AMOUNT PER SERVING: 2.3 grams of carb, 15.8
  grams of protein. NUMBER OF SERVINGS: 2.

	CHO (g)	PRO (g)
½ ounce grated Parmesan cheese (2 tablespoons)	0.5	5.9
2 tablespoons light or heavy cream	0.8	0.6
2 teaspoons mustard (Dijon type)	1.0	1.0
salt to taste (use sparingly)	0	0
freshly ground black pepper to taste	0	0
4 eggs	2.4	24.0
Total	*4.7*	*31.5*

Preheat oven to 350°F. Lightly butter or oil two 4-inch ovenproof ramekins or bowls.

Mix together the cheese, cream, mustard, salt, and freshly ground black pepper.

Crack two eggs into each ramekin. Pierce yolks with a toothpick. Bake eggs for 10 minutes. Remove from oven and spoon the cheese-mustard mixture over each egg. Return to oven and bake another 5 to 6 minutes until the eggs are done and the cheese has melted.

Variation: Microwaved Mustardy Eggs

Cover ramekins with waxed paper. Cook eggs for 2 minutes in microwave on high. Add cheese-mustard mixture. Cook for about 1 minute longer on high. (These times are approximate, since microwave ovens vary.)

Chile Pepper Eggs

Chile pepper lovers are in for a treat. This dish is a scrumptious, festive meal that would also make a lovely special-occasion breakfast or brunch. It is a cinch to toss together, while being low in carbs and high in protein.

PREPARATION TIME: 5 minutes. BAKING TIME: 17 minutes.
SERVING SIZE: ⅛ total yield. AMOUNT PER SERVING: 5.1 grams of carb, 21.7 grams of protein. NUMBER OF SERVINGS: 8.

		CHO (g)	PRO (g)
2	cans (4.5 ounces each) green, mild chile peppers, chopped	7.4	1.9
1	cup sour cream	8.0	6.4
2	ounces grated Parmesan cheese (about ½ cup)	2.0	23.8
16	eggs	9.6	96.0
	salt to taste	0	0
	freshly ground black pepper to taste	0	0
1½	cups grated cheddar cheese	2.4	42.6
16	slices of tomato (¼-inch thick)	11.2	2.7
	Total	*40.6*	*173.4*

Preheat oven to 325°F. Lightly butter or oil a 9- by 13-inch glass baking dish. Mix together the chopped chile peppers, sour cream, and Parmesan cheese and set aside.

Break the eggs into the baking dish, covering the bottom. Sprinkle with salt and freshly ground black pepper as desired. (Use salt with caution—the cheeses add plenty.) Cover the eggs with the prepared mixture of chiles, sour cream, and cheese. Bake until eggs are almost set, about 12 minutes. Remove dish from oven.

Sprinkle the dish with cheddar cheese and bake for about 5 minutes more until the cheese has melted and the eggs are done. Top with freshly sliced tomatoes and serve.

Egg and Sausage Pie

Here is an interesting change of pace from eggs with breakfast sausage links or patties. Sausage and eggs join up as a pie beneath a velvety blanket of cheese. Effort is minimal, too; it's almost a one-dish affair. For a real wake-up pie, use hot sausage. Any uncased sausage will do, though. Serve for brunch or lunch as well as breakfast.

PREPARATION TIME: 20 minutes. BAKING TIME: 13 to 15 minutes.
SERVING SIZE: ¼ pie. AMOUNT PER SERVING: 2.1 grams of carb, 24.0 grams
of protein. NUMBER OF SERVINGS: 4.

		CHO (g)	PRO (g)
1	tablespoon butter or olive oil (as desired)	0	0
8	ounces sausage (Italian mild or hot, or a mixture)	2.3	26.5
8	eggs	4.8	48.0
2	tablespoons freshly chopped parsley (or 2 teaspoons dried)	0	0
	salt to taste	0	0
	freshly ground black pepper to taste	0	0
¾	cup grated cheddar cheese, jack cheese, or combination	1.2	21.3
	Total	*8.3*	*95.8*

Preheat oven to 350°F. Lightly butter or oil a 9-inch pie pan or glass dish (or use a small or medium oval or oblong casserole dish).

Heat a skillet over medium heat. Heat butter or oil or both. Sauté the sausage in the hot fat until it is fully cooked and browned. Cool slightly so that you can touch it.

Press the sausage into the pie pan and spread it out as you would a pie crust. Break the eggs over the sausage. Sprinkle with parsley, salt (use sparingly—the sausage will add plenty), and freshly ground black pepper. Bake until the eggs are almost set, about 7 or 8 minutes. Remove from oven.

Sprinkle cheese (or cheeses) over the top of the eggs and return to oven until the eggs are done and the cheese is melted, about 6 or 7 minutes.

Florentine Baked Eggs

Another one of those quickie, delicious egg recipes that adds a bit of pizzazz to the overworked egg.

PREPARATION TIME: 10 minutes. BAKING TIME: 10 to 15 minutes.
SERVING SIZE: ½ total yield. AMOUNT PER SERVING: 2.5 grams of carb, 11.7 grams of protein. NUMBER OF SERVINGS: 2.

		CHO (g)	PRO (g)
1	tablespoon butter	0	0
1	cup thawed, well-drained, chopped frozen spinach	1.6	1.6
¼	cup whole-milk ricotta cheese	1.9	6.9
1	tablespoon grated Parmesan cheese	0.2	2.1
	salt to taste (about ½ to ¾ teaspoon)	0	0
⅛	teaspoon white pepper	0	0
⅛	teaspoon ground nutmeg	0	0
2	eggs	1.2	12.0
1	teaspoon Parmesan cheese (optional)	0.1	0.7
	Total	*5.0*	*23.3*

Preheat oven to 350°F. Lightly butter or oil two 4-inch ovenproof ramekins or bowls.

Heat a small skillet over medium heat. Add butter to skillet. When it foams (do not brown), add spinach; stir and cook quickly until the spinach is heated through, about 2 minutes.

Put the spinach in a small mixing bowl. Add the ricotta cheese, Parmesan cheese, salt, pepper, and nutmeg. Stir and divide the mixture among the two ramekins. With the back of a spoon, make a nest in the center of the spinach in each ramekin. Slide one egg onto each nest without breaking the yolk. If desired, sprinkle ½ teaspoon Parmesan cheese over each egg. Bake until eggs are set, about 10 to 15 minutes. Serve immediately.

Jalapeño Pie

Mouthwatering and sizzling, this is a breakfast to wake you up or a great lunch. This pie is easy and quick to prepare, especially if you have grated cheddar cheese on hand and chop the peppers ahead of time.

PREPARATION TIME: 15 minutes. BAKING TIME: 20 minutes.
SERVING SIZE: ½ total yield. AMOUNT PER SERVING: 2.4 grams of carb, 13.9 grams of protein. NUMBER OF SERVINGS: 6.

	CHO (g)	PRO (g)
11 ounces canned jalapeño peppers	4.1	2.9
2 tablespoons chopped pimiento	0.8	0
2 cups grated cheddar cheese	3.2	56.8
3 eggs	1.8	18.0
salt to taste	0	0
freshly ground black or white pepper to taste	0	0
¾ cup sour cream	6.0	4.8
Total	*15.9*	*82.5*

Preheat oven to 375°F. Lightly butter or oil a 9-inch pie plate. Wash, seed, and chop the jalapeño peppers.

Put the jalapeño peppers and the pimiento in the bottom of the pie pan. Sprinkle the cheese over them. In a small mixing bowl, beat the eggs lightly and beat in salt and pepper. Pour the eggs over the peppers and cheese. Bake for about 20 minutes or until done. Cool slightly. Serve with dollops of sour cream.

Berry Power Shake

You can make this irresistible, refreshing shake quickly and sip it as you get ready for the day (it's also a nice light lunch, especially on a hot day). The shake combines a mix of healthy berries with lots of protein, mostly from premium whey protein powder.

PREPARATION TIME: 5 minutes.

SERVING SIZE: 1¼ cups. AMOUNT PER SERVING: 16.4 grams of carb, 27.0 grams of protein. NUMBER OF SERVINGS: 1.

	CHO (g)	PRO (g)
1¼ cups frozen, mixed berries*	11.0	0
1 cup cold water	0	0
¼ cup cottage cheese (4% fat)	1.4	7.0
1 scoop whey protein powder	3.0	20.0
1 packet Splenda sugar substitute	1.0	0
Total	*16.4*	*27.0*

Put ingredients in a food processor or blender. Pulse to get started, then blend until smooth.

* You can mix frozen berries together or purchase them in premixed bags. (If you use fresh berries, combine them with about 1½ cups of ice cubes.) The carb count of the berries depends on the fruits. Adjust accordingly.

Choco Yogurt Cup

This is a great way to start the day—and definitely one of the speediest.

PREPARATION TIME: 3 minutes.

SERVING SIZE: 1 cup. AMOUNT PER SERVING: 17.4 grams of carb, 31.5 grams of protein. NUMBER OF SERVINGS: 1.

	CHO (g)	PRO (g)
8 ounces cup plain, whole-fat yogurt	11.4	8.5
¼ cup chocolate-flavored whey protein powder*	3.0	20.0
1 packet Splenda sugar substitute	1.0	0
1 ounce chopped pecans (about 20 halves)	2.0	3.0
Total	*17.4*	*31.5*

In a small bowl, mix or beat together yogurt and whey protein. Mix in Splenda and sprinkle with nuts.

---

* Check the label on flavored whey protein powder. The carb count may be higher. Adjust count.

4

Low-Carb Comfort Food Appetizers, Soups, Salads, and Light Lunches

A great meal usually begins with a little something to whet the appetite, but in the past those tasty bites often proved to be minefields for the low-carb dieter, because of the cracker, biscuit, puff pastry, or crust that invariably forms the presentation platform for a savory bit of salmon, a tiny wedge of cheese, or a spoonful of dip. But low-carbers need fear no more; there are chips, crackers, minirolls, tiny cocktail loaves, flaky pastry crusts, crunchy cheese biscotti, cheesy bits, and more. So you need not worry about where to put our delicious spreads and dips.

Whether you enjoy the American tradition of salad as a first course or prefer to save the greens for later in the meal, as the Europeans do, you'll have plenty of tasty choices from a quick and easy version of the classic Caesar made with our Hail of a Caesar Dressing, to savory Roasted Asparagus Salad, to the quintessential Southern experience of Wilted Lettuce Salad. If a casual luncheon or light supper is the order of the day, try one of the entree salads, such as Chicken and Avocado Salad or Cold Beef Salad. You'll find a salad here for every occasion.

You'll also find delicious options for both hot and chilled soups. If you're in the mood for something different and a little exotic, try the Peanut Soup. Or if it's just too hot to cook, how about Gazpacho or Soft Summer Soup with a warm Hearty Country Roll or a slice of Sourdough Rye? And thanks to our wide selection of low-carb breads, soup and sandwich can team up again, so what's it going to be? Chicken Noodle Soup and a tuna salad on Whole Wheat? Or Microwave Borscht with a pastrami on Gourmet Rye? The choice is, once again, yours.

Mini-Magic Rolls for Canapés

Follow the recipe for Magic Rolls in Chapter 2 on page 22. You get about 50 (plum-size) mini-rolls from one recipe. (If you do not need that many, bake them and freeze the surplus. They keep for months.) When you bake the Mini-Magic Rolls, drop the dough in the size of large grapes on the cookie sheet. You need to fit about 50 on there, so it's okay to crowd them together a bit. Bake rolls for 12 to 15 minutes in a 350°F oven or until done. Cut the rolls in half or slice off the ends before cutting them in two (that way they will have flat bottoms).

Yeast Breads for Canapés

You can choose any of the directions for yeast breads in Chapter 2 for making delightful, small slices of bread. Decide how many loaves you want to use for canapés. Let's say they require half of the recipe. Shape two bread loaves the way you always do and divide the other half of the dough into four portions. Shape each portion into a roll about 8 inches long, like a thick rope. Put them on a greased cookie sheet. You can also set the bread pans, if that is what you are using, on the cookie sheet. All can rise for the same length of time (about 60 to 75 minutes). Remove the cocktail loaves from the oven about 6 to 8 minutes earlier than the regular-size bread loaves. Cool completely. Slice the cocktail loaves thinly. Each slice should have less than 1.0 gram of carb, depending on the number of slices and the recipe.

Chive Spread

Combine 4 ounces soft cream cheese (3.2 grams of carb, 8.4 grams of protein) with 4 tablespoons (½ stick) soft butter in a blender or food processor. Add ½ cup chopped chives (0.8 gram of carb, 0.8 gram of protein). Add 1 teaspoon Worcestershire sauce (1.0 gram of carb) and salt and freshly ground black pepper to taste. TOTAL YIELD: 18 tablespoons. One tablespoon has 0.3 gram of carb and 0.5 gram of protein.

Variation: Chive Spread with Smoked Salmon

Follow the recipe for Chive Spread (above). Cover canapés generously with the spread and with slivers of smoked salmon, lox, or nova. Two ounces of smoked salmon have 11.0 grams of protein and virtually no carb.

Variation: Chive Spread with Prosciutto

Follow the recipe for Chive Spread (above). Cover canapés generously with the spread and slivers of prosciutto. Two ounces have 15.0 grams of protein and virtually no carb.

Variation: Chive Spread with Crabmeat

Follow the recipe for Chive Spread (above), but reduce chives to ¼ cup (0.4 gram of carb). Add 1 tablespoon lemon juice (1.3 grams of carb), add 1 cup cooked, well-cleaned crabmeat. Mash together. TOTAL YIELD: 2 cups. One tablespoon has 0.2 gram of carb and 1.4 grams of protein.

Sardine Spread

Even if you are not a sardine fan, here is a way to eat this marvelous and good-for-you food that may make you wonder why you never could warm up to it. Use a 3¾-ounce can of boneless and very small sardines packed in olive oil (14.0 grams of protein). Drain on paper towels and gently pat dry. Put the sardines in a small bowl and mash them with a fork. Add 1 ounce soft butter, 1 ounce soft cream cheese (0.4 gram of carb, 2.1 grams of protein), 2 tablespoons lemon juice

(2.6 grams of carb), 3 drops Tabasco sauce, salt and freshly ground pepper to taste. When you put the spread on the canapés, sprinkle them with a few snippets of parsley. TOTAL YIELD: 14 tablespoons. One tablespoon has 0.2 gram of carb and 1.2 grams of protein.

Blue Cheese Spread

Mix together 8 ounces blue cheese or Roquefort—the better the quality, the better the taste—(6.4 grams of carb, 48 grams of protein) with 4 ounces (1 stick) butter. Add salt and freshly ground pepper to taste. TOTAL YIELD: 24 tablespoons. One tablespoon has 0.3 gram of carb and 2 grams of protein.

DIPS

Chive Dip

Follow the recipe for Chive Spread on page 71. Mix in about ½ cup light cream (or the amount needed to make it the desired consistency). The cream adds 3.2 grams of carb and 2.4 grams of protein. Serve the dip at room temperature. TOTAL YIELD: 26 tablespoons. 1 tablespoon has 0.3 gram of carb and 0.4 grams of protein.

Smoked Salmon Dip

Mix together 4 ounces smoked salmon, lox, or nova (22.0 grams of protein), ¼ cup sour cream (2.0 grams of carb, 1.2 grams of protein), ¼ cup heavy cream (1.6 grams of carb, 1.2 grams of protein), 1 tablespoon minced chives, 2 teaspoons lemon juice (0.9 gram of carb), and 2 drops Tabasco sauce. Add salt and freshly ground pepper to taste. Serve the dip at room temperature. TOTAL YIELD: 16 tablespoons. One tablespoon has 0.3 gram of carb and 1.5 grams of protein.

Deviled Eggs

Here's a great way to add a bit of panache to the egg. This recipe gives you a base mix for stuffing eggs and a few suggestions—from there you can take off and add whatever you like.

PREPARATION TIME: 10 to 15 minutes.

SERVING SIZE: 1 egg. AMOUNT PER SERVING: 0.6 gram of carb, 6.0 grams of protein. NUMBER OF SERVINGS: 6.

	CHO (g)	PRO (g)
3 tablespoons butter, soft	0	0
6 hard-boiled eggs	3.6	36.0
2 tablespoons Basic Mayonnaise (page 239)	0	0
½ teaspoon Dijon-style mustard	0	0
¼ teaspoon prepared horseradish	0.2	0
salt to taste	0	0
freshly ground black pepper to taste	0	0
Total	*3.8*	*36.0*

Peel and cut eggs lengthwise once they have cooled. Scoop out yolks. Set whites on a plate and prepare the yolk mix. Put the yolks in a mixing bowl and combine the other ingredients. Mix well. For the smoothest filling, press the mixture through a sieve. For the most elegant presentation, you can put yolk mixture in a pastry tube and select an interesting, large nozzle before you fill the whites with the mixture. Otherwise, fill the eggs with a teaspoon, creating a smooth mound. For a touch of color, dust the eggs with paprika. Refrigerate until ready to use.

Variation: Deviled Eggs with Ham

Follow the recipe for Deviled Eggs (above). Add 2 ounces finely minced ham to yolk mixture and increase mustard to 1 teaspoon. This adds 2.0 grams of carb and 9.0 grams of protein to the total. A serving has 1.0 gram of carb and 6.2 grams of protein.

Variation: Deviled Eggs with Smoked Salmon

Follow the recipe for Deviled Eggs (above). Add 2 ounces finely chopped smoked salmon, lox, or nova. This adds less than 1.0 gram of carb and 11.0 grams of protein to the total. A serving has 0.8 gram of carb and 7.8 grams of protein.

Variation: Deviled Eggs with Anchovies

Follow the recipe for Deviled Eggs on page 73. Add 2 ounces finely chopped, canned anchovies. This adds no carbs and 16.4 grams of protein to the total. A serving has 8.7 grams of protein.

Variation: Deviled Eggs with Crabmeat

Follow the recipe for Deviled Eggs on page 73. Omit the mustard and horseradish. Add 1 tablespoon Tom's Low-Carb Ketchup (page 243) and 1 teaspoon lemon juice. These two ingredients add 1.3 grams of carb to total. Prepare 2 ounces cleaned and finely flaked crabmeat (11.0 grams of protein). Add the meat to the strained egg mixture. Refrigerate. Serve at room temperature. One serving has 0.9 gram of carb and 7.8 grams of protein.

Tapenade or Olive Paste

This spread may become one of your all-time favorites. It is a blend made with black olives and capers. Our version has a zesty and piquant flavor and is wonderfully low in carb per serving. Spread it on small slices of low-carb toast, rolls, bread, or crackers. Serve it as a dip. Outside of the appetizer world, spread tapenade on fish before you bake it or use it to liven up scrambled eggs for breakfast. It's quick to make and keeps well in the fridge for up to a week. You might want to have it always on hand. The recipe makes 2 cups.

PREPARATION TIME: 10 minutes.
SERVING SIZE: 1 tablespoon. AMOUNT PER SERVING: 0.7 gram of carb, 0.6 gram of protein. NUMBER OF SERVINGS: 32.

	CHO (g)	PRO (g)
2 cans black, pitted olives (11.5 ounces total dry weight)*	11.5	3.5
2 tablespoons drained capers (or more, as desired)	2.0	0
½ cup pine nuts	6.0	14.0
1 teaspoon crushed garlic in olive oil (or 2 cloves, crushed)	1.8	0.5
2 tablespoons freshly chopped parsley	0	0
salt to taste	0	0
freshly ground black pepper to taste	0	0
1 tablespoon extra-virgin olive oil	0	0
Total	*21.3*	*18.0*

Thoroughly drain olives and capers. Put all ingredients in food processor or blender. Puree to desired consistency.

* You are not limited to canned black olives. For an interesting flavor, search out a variety of olives, including black ones cured in brine that you can often find in specialty stores or delis. The most popular olive may be the Kalamata. These olives usually have a much livelier and stronger flavor. They are also usually higher in carb. Two ounces of cured olives approximate 5 ounces of canned black olives, which contain 5 grams of carb. If you use cured olives, reduce capers to 1 tablespoon.

Crunchy Cheese Biscotti

Fabulous munchies that keep virtually indefinitely. They are great as appetizers as well as anytime snacks if you're a cheese devotee. Biscotti are baked twice. Baking twice may sound like twice the work, but it's actually a pretty easy process. You bake the dough once in the form of mini-loaves, slice the loaves, and bake the slices as if they were cookies or crackers.

PREPARATION TIME: 45 minutes (requires two stages). BAKING TIME (IN TWO STAGES): around 70 minutes.

SERVING SIZE: 1 biscotti. AMOUNT PER SERVING: 0.9 gram of carb, 2.3 grams of protein. NUMBER OF SERVINGS: 60.

		CHO (g)	PRO (g)
4	ounces cream cheese, soft	3.2	8.4
4	tablespoons butter (½ stick), soft	0	0
4	egg yolks	1.2	11.2
8	ounces grated sharp cheddar cheese	3.2	56.8
¼	cup unbleached, all-purpose wheat (white) flour	23.0	3.0
1	teaspoon baking powder	1.2	0
¼	cup vital wheat gluten flour	5.6	26.0
1¼	cups whole almond meal	15.0	30.0
	Total	*52.4*	*135.4*

Once prepared, the dough will need to be refrigerated, so preheat oven to 325°F shortly before taking dough from the fridge.

Beat cream cheese, butter, and two egg yolks in the bowl of an electric mixer with a flat beater until thick, smooth, and creamy. Add the last two egg yolks and beat for another minute. Add all remaining ingredients, stirring in at slow speed or by hand. Refrigerate dough for about 30 minutes or until it can be handled without sticking.

Shape dough in four rolls about 1¾ inches in diameter and 10 inches long. Set the rolls on a nonstick, heavy-gauge metal cookie sheet and flatten them into bars about 2 inches wide and ¾ inch high. Bake for about 19 to 22 minutes or until golden.

Set oven temperature to 225°F. Put the cooled cheese bars on a cutting board and slice each bar in about 15 pieces (use a sharp, serrated knife). Set pieces upright on the cookie sheet. Bake the biscotti until they have a light golden color, about 45 minutes (always check early—do not let them turn too dark). Allow the biscotti to cool, harden, and dry completely.

Cheesy Bits

Small, rich, delectable cheese bits that should make a perfect snack for cheese lovers. One recipe will allow you to stock up for a long time. The crackers keep well and also freeze well.

PREPARATION TIME: 35 minutes. BAKING TIME: 4 sheets at about 10 minutes each or 40–50 minutes total.
SERVING SIZE: one cracker. AMOUNT PER SERVING: 0.7 gram of carb, 1.3 grams of protein. NUMBER OF SERVINGS: 90 to 95 crackers.

	CHO (g)	PRO (g)
6 tablespoons butter (¾ stick), soft	0	0
5 egg yolks	1.2	11.2
⅓ cup unbleached all-purpose wheat (white) flour	30.7	4.0
⅓ cup vital wheat gluten flour	7.5	34.7
⅓ cup unprocessed wheat bran	4.0	3.0
5 ounces grated sharp cheddar cheese (1¼ cups)	2.0	35.5
1 teaspoon baking powder	1.2	0
1 cup whole almond meal	12.0	24.0
Total	*58.6*	*112.4*

Once prepared, the dough will need to be refrigerated, so preheat oven to 325°F or 350°F shortly before taking dough from the fridge.

Beat butter and two egg yolks in the bowl of an electric mixer with a flat beater until thick, smooth, and creamy. Add the remaining egg yolks and beat some more. Stop mixer. Stir in the next five ingredients at low speed. Mix in almond meal last. Refrigerate dough for about 30 minutes or until firm enough to be handled without sticking.

Form balls the size of small grapes and put them on two large, non-stick, heavy-gauge metal cookie sheets. Flatten each cracker slightly with your fingertips.

Bake the crackers one sheet at a time, for about 8 to 10 minutes or until they have a slightly golden color with a somewhat darker color around the edge. Allow crackers to cool. They keep indefinitely at room temperature but can also be frozen.

Variation: Whole-Wheat Cheesy Bits

These give a more earthy taste to the delicate cheese crackers. Replace the wheat (white) flour with ½ cup stoneground whole-wheat flour. This adds 6.2 grams of carb to the total carb count. Carb and protein counts remain essentially unchanged.

Almond Thins

Delicate, crunchy crackers—low in carbs and bursting with almond flavor. Almond thins, served with butter, cheese, and wine are a treat to remember. No one will believe they are low-carb, but one cracker has 0.7 gram of carb. They keep indefinitely at room temperature.

PREPARATION TIME: 40 minutes. BAKING TIME: 24 minutes if you get them on 2 cookie sheets.

SERVING SIZE: one cracker. AMOUNT PER SERVING: 0.7 gram of carb, 1.0 gram of protein. NUMBER OF SERVINGS: 60 crackers.

		CHO (g)	PRO (g)
1¼	cups whole almond meal	15.0	30.0
⅓	cup crude wheat bran	4.0	2.8
⅓	cup soy protein powder	0	21.3
¼	cup unbleached, all-purpose wheat (white) flour	23.0	3.0
1	teaspoon baking powder	1.2	0
	salt to taste (about ¼ teaspoon)	0	0
	freshly ground black pepper to taste	0	0
2	tablespoons butter, soft	0	0
¼	cup cold water	0	0
1	tablespoon olive oil	0	0
2	teaspoons soy sauce	0.8	0
¼	teaspoon natural almond extract	0.2	0
	Total	*44.2*	*57.1*

Preheat oven to 300°F or 325°F.

Combine the first seven ingredients in a medium mixing bowl. Stir. Add butter in small chunks and work into the dry mix; use a pastry cutter or your fingertips.

In a separate small bowl, mix together the water, olive oil, soy sauce, and almond extract. Add the liquid mixture to the dry ingredients. Stir well. Take over by hand and work all of the ingredients into a smooth dough. (If you need a touch more liquid, add it by the teaspoon; if the dough is too moist, add a teaspoon of soy protein powder at a time.)

Shape balls about the size of olives and put them on two large, nonstick, heavy-gauge metal cookie sheets. Do not place the balls close together. Flatten each cracker slightly with your fingertips. Use the lid from a screw-top jar and press down firmly on each cracker to make them very thin. To avoid having the lid stick, put a pinch of soy protein powder (or soy flour) on it. Repeat as often as needed. Use a pastry brush to sweep all loose flour off the crackers.

Bake crackers one sheet at a time, for about 9 to 12 minutes or until lightly browned.

Yellow Squash Tea Sandwiches

A lovely addition to a light summer luncheon or brunch, a tasty different appetizer before dinner, or as part of a cocktail buffet, these cold hors d'oeuvres are utterly delicious.

PREPARATION TIME: 20 minutes
SERVING SIZE: ¹⁄₁₂ total yield. AMOUNT PER SERVING: 1.6 grams of carb, 3.8 grams of protein. NUMBER OF SERVINGS: 12.

		CHO (g)	PRO (g)
1¼	cups Basic Mayonnaise (page 239)	0	0
1	pound bacon, cooked crisp, drained thoroughly, and crumbled	0.5	40.0
1	green bell pepper, seeded and diced	3.0	0.7
72	slices of yellow crookneck squash (about 6 squash)*	15.3	4.9
	Total	*18.8*	*45.6*

In a large bowl, combine the mayonnaise, bacon, and bell pepper, mixing by hand until completely blended.

On a large sheet of waxed paper, line up the squash rounds in three rows of 12 slices. Spread the mixture, like frosting, on all slices in two of the long rows. Stack a "frosted" slice onto another "frosted" slice and top with an "unfrosted" one. Repeat this process for an additional three rows of 12 slices. You should have 24 three-tiered sandwiches when you're finished.

Arrange the tea sandwiches on a serving platter, loosely cover with plastic wrap, and refrigerate until ready to serve.

* Yellow crookneck squash, as they are known in the South, are the same as yellow zucchini or yellow summer squash.

STOCK AND BROTH

Making your own chicken stock may sound like a bother, yet it is simple to do. Instead of throwing leftover bones and skins from a chicken carcass—even that deli chicken—in the garbage, throw them in a large saucepan or stockpot, add 5 to 6 cups water, dig out a few veggies from the fridge, and add these along with some salt and pepper. Set pot to a low simmer. Once the stock simmers, remove scum that may accumulate on top, cover, and cook for several hours. Cool the stock and strain it. Put it in the fridge. Remove fat from the cooled stock, unless it was made with a natural, free-range chicken that is free from antibiotics, pesticides, and hormones. You can make a delicious chicken soup in a flash (page 81). Freeze stock it you do not plan to use it within a few days.

Many recipes call for small amounts of stock or broth. What do you do if you have no stock on hand? You can use canned beef or chicken broth. None is really great, but try to find a kind you like. Buy the fat-free kinds. Fat-free soups tend to have a slightly better flavor. Some cooks believe that low-sodium soups have the best flavor.

Extracts are not much better, and often worse, than canned soups. Again use the trial-and-error method. There is one extract, a concentrated paste, that is quite good. It is called *Better Than Bouillon* and is made by Superior Touch. One teaspoon equals 1 cup of broth and has 1.0 gram of carb. It comes in a beef and chicken base. You can use it whenever stock is called for. You might want to give it a try. Many grocery stores carry the paste. Otherwise, check the website for this product: www.superiortouch.com. It is often helpful to boost a weak stock with a touch of *Better Than Bouillon,* if you like it. You can make fairly tasty fake gravies with this concentrate, too. Clear stocks or soups vary in carbohydrate and protein content; they are low in both, generally ranging between 1.0 and 2.0 grams of carb per cup of broth and 2.0 to 4.0 grams of protein. The broth in this book contains an average of 1.0 gram of carb and 3.0 grams of protein per cup.

Chicken Soup

Make it with stock on hand (page 80) or use a combination of canned soups and extracts (page 80). Either way, soup can be served quickly. Simmer a few veggies in the stock and add chicken last. (The soup tastes good even without chicken.) In a rush, throw in a package of frozen vegetables. Serve with Magic Rolls (page 22) or Best Garlic Bread (page 26) from Chapter 2. Garlic bread takes about 15 to 20 minutes to make. This is a meal for two, a starter for four.

PREPARATION TIME: 10 minutes. COOKING TIME: 30 minutes.
SERVING SIZE: 1½ cups. AMOUNT PER SERVING: 5.5 grams of carb, 27.9 grams of protein. NUMBER OF SERVINGS: 2.

	CHO (g)	PRO (g)
2 cups chicken stock (see page 80)	2.0	6.0
1 tablespoon butter (optional)	0	0
2 tablespoons olive oil (optional)	0	0
1 cup raw, chopped broccoli	2.4	3.6
½ cup raw, chopped cauliflower (about 1-inch pieces)	3.2	2.4
½ cup chopped sweet green pepper	2.3	0
½ cup chopped zucchini	1.1	0.8
salt to taste	0	0
freshly ground black pepper to taste	0	0
1 cup diced, skinless chicken	0	43.0
Total	*11.0*	*55.8*

Put stock in a medium saucepan. Add optional butter and/or olive oil. Add vegetables. Add salt and freshly ground pepper. Simmer until vegetables are tender. This is a clear soup. If you want the soup to be slightly thicker, you can mash some veggies (right in the pot) with a potato masher or put half of the veggies (or as many as you like) in a blender or food processor and puree briefly, then return to soup. Add the diced chicken last. Reheat if needed. Adjust seasonings and serve.

Variation: Creamy Chicken Soup

Add ½ cup of heavy cream to the soup shortly before serving it. Heat through and adjust seasonings. Based on a ¼ cup serving, heavy cream adds 1.6 grams of carb and 1.2 grams of protein per serving.

Variation: Chicken Noodle Soup

Add about ⅓ cup pasta (see Chapter 6) per serving to the soup. Don't overlook the imitation pasta made from crepes. They go well with this soup and take only minutes to make. Adjust carb counts accordingly.

French Onion Soup

This traditional soup can now be returned to the low-carb menu because Magic Rolls (page 22 in Chapter 2) help bridge the gap to French bread. You can use this soup as a starter for a meal or make it a hearty lunch on chilly days.

PREPARATION TIME: 8–10 minutes. COOKING/BAKING TIME: 45 minutes.
SERVING SIZE: 1 cup. AMOUNT PER SERVING: 7.6 grams of carb, 12.7 grams of protein. NUMBER OF SERVINGS: 5 to 6.

	CHO (g)	PRO (g)
1½ cups thinly sliced onion (sweet)	16.5	2.7
2 tablespoons butter (¼ stick)	0	0
1 tablespoon Wondra flour	5.8	0.8
3½ cups stock or canned, low-carb chicken, beef, or mushroom broth (see page 80)	3.5	10.5
salt to taste	0	0
freshly ground black pepper to taste	0	0
3 Magic Rolls*	8.1	17.1
1 ounce butter	0	0
4 ounces grated Swiss cheese	4.0	32.4
Total	*37.9*	*63.5*

After this soup has finished simmering, preheat oven to 375°F. Have ready a lightly buttered, ovenproof earthenware soup bowl or deep casserole dish.

Heat 4 tablespoons butter in a heavy, medium saucepan. Add onions and cook until translucent. Add the flour and stir. Add the broth and stir. Simmer for about 30 minutes. Season with salt and freshly ground pepper. Put the soup in the ovenproof bowls.

Thinly slice the Magic Rolls, discarding the ends. Toast the slices in a toaster oven (they will brown quickly, so take care not to burn). Butter the slices and put them on top of the soup. Sprinkle cheese on top. Do not cover. Put the bowls in the oven for about 15 minutes until the cheese and Magic Roll slices look crusted over and slightly browned. Serve at once.

---

* Instead of the sliced Magic Rolls, you can use Herbed Croutons I (page 24) or gluten-free Herbed Croutons II (page 25) from Chapter 2. Use about 2 cups. Carb and protein counts remain close.

Soft Summer Soup

When it's too hot in the summer to keep the stove on for long, this creamy soup will hit the spot. Serve it with Cold Beef Salad (page 96), or Chicken and Avocado Salad (page 97). A crisp white wine, such as a pinot grigio, will set it off beautifully—or just wash it down with a large glass of refreshing herbal iced tea.

PREPARATION TIME: 10 minutes (needs 3 hours for chilling). COOKING TIME: 2 minutes.

SERVING SIZE: ⅔ cup. AMOUNT PER SERVING: 9.9 grams of carb, 6.0 grams of protein. NUMBER OF SERVINGS: 6.

		CHO (g)	PRO (g)
1	tablespoon coconut oil	0	0
½	teaspoon mustard seeds	0.4	0.5
2	large cucumbers, peeled, seeded, and sliced	10.1	3.2
4	cups buttermilk (whole)	48.0	32.0
¼	cup finely chopped fresh dill	0.1	0
1¼	teaspoons salt	0	0
¼	teaspoon celery seed	0.2	0
¼	teaspoon white pepper	0.3	0
	Total	*59.1*	*35.7*

Heat coconut oil in a small skillet over medium heat. Add mustard seeds, cover, and cook until seeds begin to pop, about 2 minutes. Remove from heat and set aside to cool slightly; drain seeds on paper towels.

In a large glass (or nonreactive) bowl, mix drained mustard seeds, cucumbers, buttermilk, dill, salt, celery seed, and white pepper. Cover and refrigerate for 3 hours. Stir hourly. Serve cold.

Gazpacho

When summer vegetables reach their peak of flavor and freshness, it's time for gazpacho. Whether you're serving it to start a meal or with a few slices of Sourdough Rye (page 36) as a light meal by itself, nothing says summer quite like it. This version—a simple blender variation—has all the flavor and none of the work of the Andalusian original.

PREPARATION TIME: 20 minutes (needs 3 hours for chilling).
SERVING SIZE: 1 cup. AMOUNT PER SERVING: 15.1 grams of carb, 6.1 grams of protein. NUMBER OF SERVINGS: 4.

	CHO (g)	PRO (g)
2 pounds fresh Roma tomatoes, seeded and quartered	32.0	6.4
1 clove garlic, minced or pressed	0.9	0
1 small red onion, peeled and quartered	5.5	0.9
1 medium cucumber, peeled, seeded, and chopped	3.5	1.4
8 ounces canned tomato juice	8.0	2.0
½ teaspoon salt	0	0
½ teaspoon black pepper	0.5	0
1 dash cayenne pepper (optional)	0	0
2 tablespoons sherry wine vinegar	0	0
1 teaspoon balsamic vinegar	0.7	0
½ cup extra-virgin olive oil	0	0
½ cup each fresh green, red, and yellow bell peppers, seeded	3.9	0.6
¼ cup scallions chopped (green and white parts)	1.2	0.0
1 cup Herbed Croutons I (page 24)	3.5	7.1
1 hard-boiled egg, chopped	0.6	6.0
Total	*60.3*	*24.4*

Put the tomatoes, garlic, red onions, cucumber, tomato juice, salt, pepper, and vinegars in a food processor or blender. Pulse until you have a chunky base (do not overprocess).

With the motor running, drizzle the olive oil in a slow stream into the blender or processor until it has been incorporated.

Pour the gazpacho base into a large bowl. Stir in the bell peppers and green onion. Cover the bowl and refrigerate until serving time. Pour or ladle about 1 cup of soup into chilled serving bowls. Garnish with Herbed Croutons and a sprinkling of chopped egg.

Microwave Borscht

An easy, quick version of the Russian classic that will leave you plenty of time to read War and Peace *or watch* Dr. Zhivago. *You can serve it hot with a Cold Beef Salad (page 96) and some warm Gourmet Rye Bread (page 36) or chill it and have it with leftover cold roast chicken for lunch. Either way, it's a meal-in-a-minute miracle.*

PREPARATION TIME: 15 minutes. COOKING TIME (MICROWAVE OVEN): 8 minutes.

SERVING SIZE: ⅙ total yield. AMOUNT PER SERVING: 7.0 grams of carb, 3.0 grams of protein. NUMBER OF SERVINGS: 6.

		CHO (g)	PRO (g)
2	teaspoons coconut oil	0	0
1	medium onion, peeled and shredded	11.0	1.8
1	can beets (16 ounces), chopped	17.3	2.9
¼	medium head green cabbage, shredded	6.3	2.8
3	cups beef broth	3.0	9.0
1	tablespoon balsamic vinegar	2.0	0
½	teaspoon salt (or to taste)	0	0
½	teaspoon freshly ground black pepper	0.5	0
3	tablespoons sour cream	1.5	1.2
2	tablespoons freshly chopped chives	0.1	0
	Total	*41.7*	*17.7*

In a microwave-safe mixing bowl large enough to hold the entire batch of soup, melt the coconut oil (about 20 seconds on high). Add the shredded onions and toss to coat with the oil. Cover loosely with waxed paper and microwave on medium power for 2 minutes.

Add the chopped beets to the onions, loosely cover with waxed paper, and microwave on medium power for another 3 minutes.

Add the shredded cabbage and beef broth to the beets and onions. Stir well, cover loosely with waxed paper, and microwave on high for 3 minutes.

Test the soup. The vegetables should be cooked but not mushy. If necessary, cook a bit longer in 20-second intervals, testing between each interval. When done, season with the balsamic vinegar, salt, and pepper.

Spoon into bowls, top with a dollop of sour cream, a sprinkling of fresh chives, and serve.

Peanut Soup

When you're in the mood for something exotic, treat yourself and your guests to this unusual soup. It's high in protein for a legume-based soup but reasonably modest in carbs; all you need is a salad, some warm Black Soybean Bread (page 29) and butter or Gourmet Rye Bread (page 36). Start a pot of hot green tea to make a meal. If you're really protein hungry, serve with a couple of grilled chicken or beef skewers for good measure. This recipe can be multiplied easily— limited only by the size of your soup kettle.

PREPARATION TIME: 20 minutes. COOKING TIME: 20 minutes
SERVING SIZE: ¼ total yield. AMOUNT PER SERVING: 12.0 grams of carb, 15.0 grams of protein. NUMBER OF SERVINGS: 4.

		CHO (g)	PRO (g)
2	tablespoons butter	0	0
1	rib celery, finely chopped	0.8	0.3
5	scallions (green and white parts), minced	5.0	0
1	tablespoon soy flour	1.4	1.9
4	cups chicken broth	4.0	12.0
½	cup chunky peanut butter (no-sugar-added variety)	20.0	32.0
1½	cups whole milk	16.0	13.5
1	teaspoon black pepper	1.0	0
1	teaspoon salt (optional)	0	0
1	sprinkle paprika	0	0
	Total	*48.2*	*59.7*

In a large soup kettle or stockpot, melt the butter over low heat. Add the celery and onion and sauté until translucent and soft but not browned. Add the soy flour and cook for 2 to 3 minutes, stirring constantly. Gradually add the chicken broth, stirring constantly to keep the mixture smooth. When all the broth is incorporated, bring it to a boil, then blend in the peanut butter.

Reduce heat and simmer the soup for about 12 minutes, uncovered. Stir occasionally.

Add the milk and black pepper and stir well to combine. Heat through—about 5 minutes—but do not let the soup boil. Taste for seasoning; add salt only if it's needed. Ladle soup into bowls, sprinkle with a dash of paprika, and serve.

Zuppa Toscano

When you're in the mood for a hearty soup, this is the one: filling, rich, and savory. Add a tossed salad and a few warm slices of Best Garlic Bread (page 26) and you're done. The recipe can be multiplied easily for a bigger crowd.

PREPARATION AND COOKING TIME: 30 minutes.
SERVING SIZE: 8 ounces. AMOUNT PER SERVING: 5.9 grams of carb,
   24.3 grams of protein. NUMBER OF SERVINGS: 4.

		CHO (g)	PRO (g)
2	tablespoons olive oil	0	0
1	clove garlic, minced	0.9	0.2
1	small yellow onion, chopped	5.3	0.8
8	ounces spicy sausage links, cut into		
	½-inch pieces	2.4	44.7
12	ounces bacon, cut into 1-inch pieces	0.3	30.0
1	cup sliced white mushrooms	1.5	1.1
4	cups fresh baby spinach leaves	1.0	3.4
3	cups chicken broth	3.0	9.0
1	teaspoon salt	0	0
1	teaspoon black pepper	1.0	0
1	cup half and half	8.1	8.1
	Total	*23.5*	*97.3*

In a stockpot, heat the olive oil. Add the garlic and the onions and sauté until onions are translucent. Do not allow to brown or burn. Add the sausage and bacon and brown fully, stirring often to prevent burning or sticking.

Add the mushrooms, stirring often, and cook until soft.

Add the spinach and allow it to cook down.

Add the chicken broth, salt, and pepper and bring to a boil.

Turn down the heat to simmer, add the half and half, and heat through. Serve hot.

Roasted Asparagus Salad

Delicious, nutritious, low in starch and high in protein, asparagus is a low-carb dieter's staple. It's enjoyable in many ways, but this easy, simple salad really lets the distinctive asparagus taste come through loud and clear. Pair it with roasted poultry, grilled meats, baked fish, or just about any simply prepared entree. You could even put it, still warm, over a bowl of pasta (see Chapter 6 for pasta recipes) with a light cream sauce for a tasty, quick supper.

PREPARATION TIME: 8 to 10 minutes. BAKING TIME: 8 minutes.
SERVING SIZE: ⅛ total yield. AMOUNT PER SERVING: 3.5 grams of carb, 6.0 grams of protein. NUMBER OF SERVINGS: 8.

		CHO (g)	PRO (g)
2½	pounds fresh asparagus (with thick stems)	24.3	24.4
3	tablespoons plus 1 teaspoon olive oil	0	0
½	teaspoon salt	0	0
¾	teaspoon white pepper	1.0	0
2	teaspoons fresh lemon juice	1.0	0
2	ounces Parmigiano Reggiano	2.0	23.6
	Total	*28.3*	*48.0*

Preheat oven to 500°F.

Wash asparagus, and pat dry. Snap or cut woody stem ends, leaving only the tender portion. Gently peel the bottom third with a vegetable peeler if necessary. Slice each spear on the diagonal into about three pieces.

In a large bowl, combine the olive oil, salt, and white pepper. Add the cut asparagus and toss to coat evenly. Set aside and allow asparagus to marinate in this mixture for about 8 to 10 minutes at room temperature.

When marinated, transfer the asparagus to a nonstick, heavy-gauge metal baking sheet, spread out in a single layer, and roast for about 8 minutes, shaking several times during the roasting period to cook evenly and prevent sticking. When roasted, remove from oven and allow to cool to room temperature.

When ready to serve, sprinkle lemon juice over the roasted asparagus and toss to coat. Divide the asparagus evenly among eight plates. Using a cheese slicer or vegetable peeler, slice thin curls of the Parmigiano Reggiano atop the asparagus.

Avocado Slaw

You could think of this Southwestern spin on an old Southern favorite as coleslaw meets guacamole. It pairs well with many of the Mexican dishes you'll find in Chapter 6 as well as such picnic and cookout staples as burgers, hot dogs, ribs, and barbecued chicken. We think of it as Olé! Slaw.

PREPARATION TIME: 20 minutes.
SERVING SIZE: ¹⁄₁₀ total yield. AMOUNT PER SERVING: 6.1 grams of carb, 3.3 grams of protein. NUMBER OF SERVINGS: 10.

		CHO (g)	PRO (g)
4	small Haas avocados, peeled and seeded	13.9	14.6
3	tablespoons fresh lime juice (about 1½ limes)	3.9	0
8	ounces sour cream	8.0	6.4
1	clove garlic, pressed	0.9	0
½	teaspoon cumin	0.4	0
1	teaspoon salt	0	0
½	teaspoon ground red chile pepper	0.2	0
8	cups prepackaged coleslaw salad mix*	23.5	8.2
1½	cups chopped scallions (green and white parts)	7.2	2.7
1	small red bell pepper, diced	3.3	0.7
	Total	*61.3*	*32.6*

Chop one of the avocados coarsely and drizzle 1 tablespoon of lime juice over the pieces, tossing gently to coat. Cover and set aside. Chop and mash (a fork and a shallow bowl work well for this procedure) the other three avocados with the remainder of the lime juice. Add the sour cream, garlic, cumin, salt, and red chile pepper to the mashed avocados and combine well.

Put the coleslaw salad mix in a large bowl, top with the mashed avocado mixture, and toss to combine evenly. Fold in the chunks of chopped avocado, the green onion, and the red bell pepper. Toss gently. Serve immediately or cover tightly with plastic wrap placed directly on the avocado slaw to prevent air from reaching it and refrigerate until ready to use.

---

* If you can't find prepackaged coleslaw salad mix in your grocery store, you can simply wash and shred a small head or two of cabbage to make 7 cups and add 1 cup of shredded carrot to it.

Coleslaw Supreme

When you yearn for the sizzle of a summer cookout and can almost smell the ribs cooking on the grill, it's time to start shredding the cabbage for a big batch of cole slaw. Pair it up with some Deviled Eggs (page 73), Best Garlic Bread (page 26), and iced tea and you're ready to invite all the neighbors for a feast . . . Southern style.

PREPARATION TIME: 20 to 25 minutes.
SERVING SIZE: ¹/₁₂ total yield. AMOUNT PER SERVING: 3.4 grams of carb, 1.3 grams of protein. NUMBER OF SERVINGS: 12.

		CHO (g)	PRO (g)
2	medium carrots, shredded	10.2	1.4
2	cups Basic Mayonnaise (page 239)	0	0
½	teaspoon dry mustard	0.5	0.5
½	teaspoon white pepper	0.5	0
¼	cup champagne vinegar (or other white vinegar)	0.5	0
2	tablespoons fresh lemon juice (about 1 lemon)	2.6	0
1	teaspoon salt (or to taste)	0	0
½	teaspoon celery seed	0.6	0
3	medium heads green cabbage, shredded (about 12 cups)	26.4	13.0
	Total	*41.3*	*14.9*

In a large bowl, combine the mayonnaise, mustard, pepper, vinegar, lemon juice, salt, and celery seed. Mix well. Add the cabbage and toss to coat evenly with the slaw dressing. Cover and chill until time to serve (or serve immediately if the ribs are done!).

Wilted Lettuce Salad

Nothin' says lovin' like a wilted lettuce salad. This savory combination of textures and tastes is quintessentially Southern. Serve it with Southern Fried Chicken (page 111), Mock Mashed Potatoes (page 218), Crookneck Casserole (page 230), and warm Magic Rolls (page 22) with butter and it'll carry you back to ole Virginia before you can say Mason-Dixon.

PREPARATION TIME: 10 minutes. COOKING TIME: 8 to 10 minutes.
SERVING SIZE: ¼ total yield. AMOUNT PER SERVING: 0.6 gram of carb, 2.4 grams of protein. NUMBER OF SERVINGS: 4.

	CHO (g)	PRO (g)
2 cups freshly chopped lettuce (any kind)	1.8	1.5
4 strips bacon, cut into 1-inch pieces	0.1	7.9
¼ cup apple cider vinegar	0.6	0
Total	*2.5*	*9.4*

Put the lettuce in a heatproof salad bowl and refrigerate until you're ready to make the hot dressing—just moments before you're planning to serve the salad. Then remove from the refrigerator and keep at hand near the stove.

Fry the bacon pieces—traditionally in a cast-iron skillet—until they are crisp and brown, but do not allow them to burn. Slowly and carefully add the vinegar to the skillet—it may spatter and hiss, so take care not to get burned. Heat the mixture to the boiling point, stirring constantly.

Immediately pour the hot bacon dressing over the greens, toss quickly to coat the lettuce evenly, and serve right away.

Note: You can substitute baby spinach for the lettuce for a different but equally luscious wilted salad. In that case, you might want to throw on a tablespoon or two of finely chopped hard-boiled egg and a few sliced fresh mushrooms for a negligible increase in carb grams per serving.

Winter Radish Salad

So simple, so tasty, and so low in carb that you'll want to serve this crunchy salad again and again, especially in the fall and winter when tomatoes usually taste like cardboard. This little salad makes a great starter or accompaniment to chicken, pork, or fish dishes. The recipe can be multiplied easily for big groups or for buffet suppers.

PREPARATION TIME: 20 minutes.
SERVING SIZE: ⅙ total yield. AMOUNT PER SERVING: 2.7 grams of carb, 1.2 grams of protein. NUMBER OF SERVINGS: 6.

	CHO (g)	PRO (g)
2 cups sliced radishes	4.6	1.4
½ cup sour cream	4.0	3.2
1 teaspoon Dijon-style mustard	0.5	0.5
½ teaspoon salt (or to taste)	0	0
½ teaspoon white pepper	0.5	0
2 cups freshly torn or shredded lettuce (any kind)	1.2	1.6
Total	*10.8*	*6.7*

In a bowl large enough to hold the dressing and radishes, combine the sour cream, mustard, salt, and white pepper. Fold in the radishes and toss to coat.

Divide the shredded lettuce equally among six salad plates. Top each bed of lettuce with the dressed radish mixture and serve immediately.

Sour Cream Cucumber Salad

Modest on carbs but long on flavor, this salad goes well with grilled sausages, steaks, chicken, or fish. Prepare this easy salad the day you plan to serve it (otherwise the cucumbers will soften, become mushy, and lose the pleasant crunch that helps make this salad appealing). The recipe can be multiplied easily.

PREPARATION TIME: 1¼ hours (largely unattended).

SERVING SIZE: ⅙ total yield. AMOUNT PER SERVING: 4.0 grams of carb, 2.4 grams of protein. NUMBER OF SERVINGS: 6.

		CHO (g)	PRO (g)
1	teaspoon salt	0	0
2	tablespoons tarragon vinegar	0.3	0
1	cup sour cream	8.0	6.4
1	teaspoon celery seeds	0.6	0
2	tablespoons chopped scallions (green and white parts)	0.6	0
3	medium cucumbers	10.9	3.4
6	cups freshly torn or shredded lettuce (any kind)	3.6	4.8
	Total	*24.0*	*14.6*

In a large mixing bowl, dissolve the salt in the vinegar. Add the sour cream and stir until smooth. Add the celery seeds and the chopped scallion to the sour cream mixture and set aside.

Peel cucumbers and slice them very thinly. Combine the sliced cucumbers with the sour cream mixture, turning over and over to evenly coat all the slices with the dressing. Cover and chill no more than 1 hour.

When ready to serve, place a cup of freshly torn lettuce on each of six plates and top with sour cream–cucumber mixture.

Three-Bean Salad

The trio is made up of crunchy green beans, black soybeans, and a handful of garbanzo beans. Give them even more life with some chopped onion. Mix with extra virgin olive oil and a good vinegar—and here is a nice side to go with almost any meal. Or have the salad for a light supper with warm Best Garlic Bread (page 26). This salad can be assembled quickly; if you are in a hurry, substitute canned green beans for the freshly cooked ones.

PREPARATION TIME: 20 minutes. (Refrigerate for 1 hour or longer).
SERVING SIZE: ⅙ total yield. AMOUNT PER SERVING: 6.4 grams of carb, 5.8 grams of protein. NUMBER OF SERVINGS: 6.

		CHO (g)	PRO (g)
2	cups green beans (or one 15-ounce can cut green beans)	8.0	4.0
½	cup drained and rinsed canned garbanzo beans	11.0	5.0
15	ounces organic black soybeans, drained and rinsed	11.2	24.2
½	cup finely chopped onion	5.5	0.9
½	cup finely chopped celery	1.2	0.5
1	clove garlic, pressed	0.9	0
1	tablespoon freshly chopped parsley	0	0
¼	cup extra-virgin olive oil	0	0
¼	cup red wine vinegar	0	0
	salt to taste	0	0
	freshly ground black pepper to taste	0	0
½	packet Splenda sugar substitute (or as needed)	0.5	0
	Total	*38.3*	*34.6*

Clean and trim green beans; cut in 1-inch pieces. Steam until barely tender. Cool a bit. Combine with the garbanzo beans and black soybeans in a mixing or serving bowl. Add onion, celery, garlic, and parsley to the beans. Mix together oil, vinegar, salt, pepper, and Splenda. Pour over bean mixture. Stir to coat well.

Refrigerate for 1 hour or longer. Stir periodically to distribute flavors. Allow to sit at room temperature for a while before serving.

Fresh Beet Salad

The earthy taste of beets highlights this simple starter. If you like beets, you'll be a goner for this salad. You'll want to save time by roasting extra beets so that you can have them on hand to accompany chicken, steak, roast pork, or game dishes. Or save a few for the Microwave Borscht (page 85).

PREPARATION TIME: 15 minutes. BAKING TIME: 1 hour.
SERVING SIZE: ¼ total yield. AMOUNT PER SERVING: 8.2 grams of carb, 2.6 grams of protein. NUMBER OF SERVINGS: 4.

		CHO (g)	PRO (g)
1	pound fresh beets	30.1	7.3
2	tablespoons sherry or red wine vinegar	0.2	0
½	teaspoon salt	0	0
1	tablespoon freshly chopped chives	0	0
1	tablespoon extra-virgin olive oil	0	0
4	cups freshly torn salad greens	2.4	3.2
	Total	*32.7*	*10.5*

Preheat oven to 350°F.

Cut green tops from the beets; do not trim the root ends. Wash beets well, scrubbing with a vegetable brush if necessary. Pat dry.

Put the beets in a covered baking dish; add approximately ½ cup warm water to the dish. Cover and bake until you can easily pierce the beets with a fork, about 1 hour.

Remove beets from the oven and allow them to cool. When cool, trim both ends and slip off the skins under cool running water. Cut the beets in half, then slice thinly. Cut the slices in half again. Set aside. (You can roast the beets, cool them, and seal them in an airtight bag in the refrigerator for a couple of days. You can also proceed with the cleaning, slicing, etc., and put the prepped pieces in an airtight bag for a day or two, to dress and assemble the salad at a later point.)

In a small bowl, whisk together the vinegar, salt, and chives. Then drizzle in the olive oil slowly as you constantly whisk to combine. Pour this vinaigrette over the beets and toss gently to coat evenly. Cover and chill the beets for at least 10 minutes. (You can chill for several hours if needed.)

When ready to serve, divide the freshly torn salad greens among four plates. Put the beet mixture on each lettuce bed and serve.

Cold Beef Salad

On a warm spring or summer day, this cold entree salad makes the perfect easy luncheon or alfresco supper. Serve it with a couple of slices of Best Garlic Bread (page 26) and a full-bodied red wine. Add some fresh berries and whipped cream for dessert. The recipe is a great way to use leftover roast beef or steak. It is easy to make in small quantities.

PREPARATION TIME: 20 minutes.

SERVING SIZE: ⅛ total yield. AMOUNT PER SERVING: 1.4 grams of carb, 16.9 grams of protein. NUMBER OF SERVINGS: 8.

		CHO (g)	PRO (g)
1	cup Basic Vinaigrette (page 236)	0	0
8	cups freshly torn red-leaf lettuce	4.8	6.4
4	cups cooked beefsteak strips	0	127.0
¼	cup green bell pepper strips	1.2	0
¼	cup red bell pepper strips	1.2	0
½	cup chopped scallion (green and white parts)	2.4	0.9
¼	cup chopped fresh flat-leaf (Italian) parsley	0.5	0.5
1	teaspoon black pepper	1.0	0
	Total	*11.1*	*134.8*

Put freshly torn lettuce into a large bowl. Add ¼ cup of the dressing and coat evenly and lightly.

Combine beef, green and red pepper strips, and onion in a mixing bowl. Add ¾ cup (the remainder) of the dressing and toss well.

Put the red-leaf lettuce on eight plates. Top each lettuce bed with the beef mixture (about ½ cup) and garnish with the chopped parsley and pepper.

Chicken and Avocado Salad

When you cook chicken breasts, it's a good idea to cook a couple of extra halves so that on a warm summer evening you can make this delicious entree salad. (If you do need to roast the chicken, directions are given.) All you need is a bottle of chilled Sauvignon Blanc and a warm loaf of Sourdough Rye (page 36) for a meal fit for royalty.

PREPARATION TIME: 20 minutes (assuming you have roasted chicken on hand, if not, add about 40 minutes for roasting time).

SERVING SIZE: ½ total yield. AMOUNT PER SERVING: 8.1 grams of carb, 35.8 grams of protein. NUMBER OF SERVINGS: 2.

	CHO (g)	PRO (g)
2 boneless, skinless chicken breast halves, roasted and diced	0	53.4
1 tablespoon lemon juice	1.3	0
½ teaspoon salt	0	0
½ teaspoon freshly ground black pepper	0.5	0
4 tablespoons olive oil	0	0
2 medium Haas avocados, peeled and diced (ripe and soft)	7.0	7.3
4 cups freshly torn lettuce (any kind)	2.4	3.2
1 bunch watercress (about ¾ cup)	0.0	0.6
1 medium tomato, quartered	4.4	1.1
2 tablespoons grated Parmesan cheese	0.5	5.9
Total	*16.1*	*71.5*

If you need to roast the chicken, preheat oven to 350°F and oil or butter a roasting pan. Rub the chicken breasts with a bit of olive oil, sprinkle with salt and pepper, and roast for about 35 minutes. Check in a thick portion of the meat for doneness—the juices should run clear. If not, roast for another 5 to 10 minutes. Cool and dice.

In a small bowl, combine the lemon juice, salt, and pepper. Add the olive oil in a slow stream, whisking all the while, until all 4 tablespoons have been incorporated smoothly. Put the avocado in the dressing and toss to coat and prevent browning.

Put the salad greens in a large salad bowl and pour the dressing and avocados over them. Toss to coat lightly and evenly. Add the diced chicken and toss gently again.

Divide the mixture between two salad plates. Arrange two tomato quarters on each plate and top with Parmesan cheese before serving.

Crabby Luncheon Special

This light crab salad makes the perfect luncheon plate for a warm summer day. Invite a couple of friends over; open a bottle of crisp Sauvignon Blanc or pinot blanc to accompany the salad and good conversation. You can have the salad ready except for the assembly. For dessert, serve cooled whole seasonal fruits, such as peaches or plums. Double or triple the recipe for a bigger group.

PREPARATION TIME: 25 minutes.
SERVING SIZE: ½ cup. AMOUNT PER SERVING: 4.3 grams of carb, 20.0 grams of protein. NUMBER OF SERVINGS: 3.

	CHO (g)	PRO (g)
½ cup Basic Mayonnaise (page 239)	0	0
1 tablespoon chopped fresh parsley	0	0
1 teaspoon dry mustard	0.5	0.9
1 teaspoon prepared horseradish	1.0	0
1 hard-boiled egg, chopped	0.6	6.0
2 tablespoons chopped pimiento	0.8	0
½ teaspoon lemon juice	0.2	0
1 cup fresh lump crabmeat, picked for shells	0	31.5
3 cups freshly torn lettuce (any kind)	1.8	2.4
3 hard-boiled eggs, peeled and quartered	1.8	18.0
1 medium tomato, cut in 6 wedges	4.3	1.0
3 tablespoons sliced black olives	2.0	0
Total	*13.0*	*59.8*

In a medium-size mixing bowl, combine the mayonnaise, parsley, dry mustard, and horseradish. Add the chopped egg, pimiento, and lemon juice. Stir to combine. Add the crabmeat and stir to combine. Cover and refrigerate for at least 1 hour to allow flavors to blend.

To assemble the salads, put 1 cup of lettuce on each plate and top with ½ cup crab salad. Arrange the quartered eggs and tomato wedges around the salad and sprinkle 1 tablespoon of sliced black olives over each plate. Pass around Blue Cheese Dressing (page 241) or Basic Vinaigrette (page 236) to drizzle over the salad greens, if desired. Calculate the additional carbs if you use dressing.

Shrimp and Deviled Egg Salad

This salad is perfect for dinner on a hot summer day when nobody feels much like cooking. You can prepare everything ahead and simply fix the individual serving plates at mealtime. Sometimes you can get cooked shrimp that have not been previously frozen. They deliver the best flavor. If you buy frozen shrimp, buy them completely frozen, not partially thawed (as from a display tray). If possible, taste or smell a sample shrimp before you buy. They should not smell. This recipe is for two but can be multiplied as needed. For bigger appetites, you may want to increase the amount of shrimp slightly.

PREPARATION TIME: 25 minutes.
SERVING SIZE: ½ total yield. AMOUNT PER SERVING: 10.1 grams of carb, 42.9 grams of protein. NUMBER OF SERVINGS: 2.

		CHO (g)	PRO (g)
10	ounces cooked shrimp meat (salad shrimp)	0	59.3
¾	cup milk (for marinade—to be discarded)	0	0
1½	cups freshly torn iceberg or romaine lettuce	0.9	1.5
4	Deviled Eggs (page 73)	2.8	24.0
2	medium-sized ripe tomatoes, cut in wedges	8.0	1.0
2	lemon wedges	1.3	0
1	tablespoon chopped fresh parsley	0	0
6	tablespoons Low-Carb Cocktail Sauce (page 244)	7.2	0
	Total	*20.2*	*85.8*

Put the shrimp (fresh or frozen) in the milk for about 1 to 2 hours before serving time. Drain and pat completely dry with lots of paper towels upon removal.

To assemble the salad, put the bed of lettuce leaves on two plates. Put the shrimp in the center. Surround the shrimp with deviled eggs, tomato wedges, and lemon wedges. Sprinkle the salads with the parsley. Top shrimp with cocktail sauce.

5

LOW-CARB COMFORT FOOD POULTRY, MEAT, GAME, AND SEAFOOD ENTREES

It's certainly not news that poultry, meat, game, and seafood are low-carb foods, but what you'll find here are recipes designed to free you from the yet-another-baked-chicken-breast- or hamburger-patty-for-dinner blues that has traditionally plagued low-carb dieters. For instance, how long has it been since you experienced the taste of real Southern Fried Chicken without a pang of guilt? Remember the crunch of biting into the crispy breaded crust and the savory softness of the tender, juicy meat beneath it? Or what about tender chicken baked in a rich sweet-and-sour sauce? Or Chicken Schnitzel? If you've been missing these comforting dishes in an effort to curb your carb intake, we've got a treat in store for you in this chapter. They're back, low in carb and rich in flavor—just like Grandma used to make . . . almost.

When the leaves start to turn, the weather begins to cool, and you long for the comfort of a roasted chicken, turkey, or duck with all the trimmings, get ready to dig in. All you'll have to decide is which savory dressing sounds best.

If it's red meat you crave, you'll find Stuffed Blue Cheese Patties—a savory steak, egg, and spinach combination—Veal Stew, Caraway Beef Stew, and Rosemary Leg of Lamb, along with a selection of savory casseroles—all tasty and interesting twists on some of your old favorites. But the big news is that you'll also find some meat dishes you'd never have believed you could eat while keeping your low-carb commitment. How about Breaded Pork Chops? Bet you thought you'd never see those on a low-carb plate. With a big side of Mock Mashed Potatoes (page 218 in Chapter 7) and low-carb Pan Gravy (page 111), you won't believe it's not Sunday dinner at Granny's.

And if the exotic intrigues you, you'll find some amazingly easy gourmet recipes for game dishes using buffalo, venison, and ostrich.

Since game meats offer the best of protein nutrition—high-quality lean protein and good-quality fats—it makes sense to treat yourself to them when you can, especially since they're commercially available nationwide.

Traditionally, the low-carb menu for fish and shellfish reached its limit with grilled, broiled, or sautéed offerings—all of which are delicious and good for you. We've included some of these simple staple recipes here, but what all low-carbers miss are those forbidden cooking methods—in short, we all miss the breading on fish fillets, shrimp, and calamari. But no more! Thanks to the miracle of Bread Crumbs I (page 251) and gluten-fee Bread Crumbs II (page 26) in Chapter 2, breaded fish and shellfish are no longer forbidden—they're just one more tasty option in your low-carb recipe file.

But once you've exhausted your pent-up longing for breaded fish, we thought you might want something a bit different. How about Tuna Crunch, a savory pan-fried burger that you can sandwich in a low-carb burger bun, or a Baked Tuna Burger? Or if you've missed the creamy comfort of casseroles hot from the oven, try Tuna Casserole, Easy Salmon Casserole, or the best Scampi you've ever tasted. Round off your meal with a salad and a loaf of warm Sourdough Rye (page 36), of course.

Chicken Schnitzel

The chicken breasts are pounded very thin, then breaded and pan-fried. This is a special treat. You can use Bread Crumbs I (page 25) or gluten-free Bread Crumbs II (page 26) in Chapter 2. As you pound the breasts, they become quite large. If you plan to cook several schnitzels, you may want to preheat the oven and keep the schnitzels that are done warm until the rest catch up.

PREPARATION AND COOKING TIME: 50 minutes.

SERVING SIZE: 1 schnitzel. AMOUNT PER SERVING: 4.8 grams of carb, 41.8 grams of protein. NUMBER OF SERVINGS: 2.

	CHO (g)	PRO (g)
2 eggs, lightly beaten	1.2	12.0
¾ cup Bread Crumbs I (page 25)	8.4	17.1
4 tablespoons grated Parmesan cheese (optional)	1.0	11.9
salt to taste	0	0
freshly ground black pepper to taste	0	0
2 boneless, skinless chicken breast halves	0	54.4
3 (or more) tablespoons coconut or olive oil	0	0
3 (or more) tablespoons butter	0	0
parsley sprigs	0	0
4 lemon wedges (garnish)	0	0
Total	*10.6*	*95.4*

Pour the beaten eggs onto a large plate. Put the bread crumbs and optional cheese on another plate. Add salt and freshly ground pepper to the crumbs.

Remove visible fat from the chicken breasts; wash and pat very dry with paper towels. Slide each breast into a plastic (tie-type) bag. Do not tie bag. Place on a cutting board. With a meat mallet (smooth side), pound the chicken breasts very thin, to about ¼ inch. The pieces become quite large. If you like, you can cut them in half.

Dip the chicken pieces first in the beaten egg, then in the bread crumbs. Coat well. Place coated pieces on a platter.

Heat oil and butter in one or two large, heavy skillets over medium-low heat (more on the low side). Add the breaded chicken to the hot fat and brown lightly on both sides. Reduce heat and cook until done, about 4 to 5 minutes on each side. Low-carb bread crumbs tend to darken more quickly than regular bread crumbs. Keep the heat a notch lower than you would normally and check the underside of the chicken after a minute or two. If the breading is getting too dark, reduce heat further. Serve schnitzels garnished with parsley and lemon wedges.

Angel Wings

When you serve these wings, your guests will proclaim them the best wings they ever tasted. And these savory, cheesy wings are so easy, you'll be tempted to serve them often. They're great as a meal with a salad or coleslaw but just as good as a snack or at a cocktail buffet. Why not make a big batch for a game-day party?

PREPARATION TIME: 20 minutes. BAKING TIME: 1 hour.
SERVING SIZE: 5 wings. AMOUNT PER SERVING: 3.0 grams of carb, 39.0 grams of protein. NUMBER OF SERVINGS: 4.

		CHO (g)	PRO (g)
20	chicken wings	0	83.8
1½	cups grated Parmesan cheese	6.0	71.4
1	teaspoon dried chopped parsley	0	0
2	teaspoons garlic powder	4.6	1.0
1	teaspoon white pepper	1.2	0
1	cup butter, melted	0	0
	Total	*11.8*	*156.2*

Wash chicken wings and pat dry with paper towels.

Preheat oven to 350°F. Lightly grease an ovenproof baking dish (or broiler pan) large enough to accommodate all the wings with olive oil or coconut oil.

In a wide, shallow bowl, combine the cheese, parsley, garlic powder, and white pepper, mixing well.

Dip wings first in melted butter, then in the cheese and spice mixture. Arrange them in the baking dish and bake uncovered for 1 hour. Serve hot.

Fiery Chicken

Some like 'em hot! And if you're one who does, these spicy chicken breasts have your name on them. You can vary the heat by adjusting the amount of Tabasco you use—and at virtually zero carbs per teaspoon, you can crank up the heat to high and make barely a ripple in your overall carb intake! Serve this dish with a colorful tossed salad of lettuces and fresh veggies (something cool to balance the heat) and a slice or two of delicious low-carb Garlic Bread (page 26). Double the batch for a bigger crowd or for bigger appetites.

PREPARATION TIME: 15 minutes. BAKING TIME: 50 minutes to 1 hour.
SERVING SIZE: 1 breast. AMOUNT PER SERVING: 2.2 grams of carb, 31.6 grams of protein. NUMBER OF SERVINGS: 4.

		CHO (g)	PRO (g)
4	split chicken breasts with skin and bones	0	120.0
1	cup sour cream	8.0	6.4
2	teaspoons Tabasco sauce	0.1	0
½	teaspoon celery salt	0	0
½	teaspoon black pepper	0.5	0
	Total	*8.6*	*126.4*

Preheat oven to 350°F. Butter or oil an ovenproof baking pan large enough to accommodate the chicken pieces.

Wash chicken and pat dry with paper towels. (*Optional:* For the tastiest, juiciest chicken, wash the night before, and while still wet, sprinkle liberally with Kosher or coarse salt, cover tightly, and refrigerate overnight. Rinse well and pat dry, then proceed with the recipe below.) Place chicken in greased baking dish.

In a cup or small bowl, combine the sour cream, Tabasco sauce, celery salt, and pepper. Spread this cream mixture evenly over the chicken. Cover baking dish with foil or a tight-fitting lid and bake for 50 minutes to 1 hour. Serve immediately.

Touch of India Chicken

Not only can chicken be changed in surprising ways, but it can be done with little effort. This dish tastes as if you had cooked an elaborate meal. Cauliflower cooks alongside the chicken; turmeric and ginger enliven both. Serve over Supreme Pasta (page 172) or other pastas from Chapter 6. Magic Rolls (page 22) from Chapter 2 are always a reliable standby.

PREPARATION AND COOKING TIME: 45 minutes.
SERVING SIZE: ¼ total yield. AMOUNT PER SERVING: 8.9 grams of carb, 32.7 grams of protein. NUMBER OF SERVINGS: 4.

		CHO (g)	PRO (g)
16	ounces cleaned, broken cauliflower florets (ready to cook)	12.8	9.6
4	boneless, skinless chicken breast halves	0	108.8
3	tablespoons olive or coconut oil	0	0
2	tablespoons butter	0	0
	salt to taste	0	0
	freshly ground black pepper to taste	0	0
½	cup chopped onion	5.5	0.9
2	cloves garlic, minced (or ½ teaspoon garlic powder)	1.8	0
½	teaspoon ground turmeric (or to taste)	0.5	0
2	teaspoons ground ginger (or to taste)	2.2	0
1½	cups stock or broth (see page 80)	1.5	4.5
2	tablespoons tomato paste	5.0	2.0
1	cup heavy cream	6.4	4.8
	freshly chopped or dried parsley (small amount)	0	0
1	tablespoon olive or coconut oil, if needed	0	0
	Total	*35.7*	*130.6*

Parboil or steam cauliflower in a small amount of water for about 5 minutes; drain.

Remove visible fat from chicken. Wash chicken and pat very dry with paper towels. Cut each breast in bite-size pieces.

Heat a large, heavy skillet over medium heat. Add oil and butter. When the butter is bubbly (do not brown), add the chicken and brown quickly on both sides (about 1 minute per side). Sprinkle lightly with salt and pepper. Remove chicken from skillet and set aside.

Add a little more oil to skillet if needed. Sauté onion until soft. Add garlic, turmeric, and ginger. Stir for 1 minute. Add broth and tomato paste. Stir until smooth. Add cauliflower and chicken pieces. Reduce heat. Simmer chicken and cauliflower very slowly for about 5 minutes. Add cream. Simmer for 10 minutes or until chicken is done, stirring several times. When the chicken is ready, the sauce will be reduced and nice and thick (if it gets too thick, add a little broth). Adjust seasoning, sprinkle with parsley, and serve.

Southern Fried Chicken with Pan Gravy

Southern fried chicken, with delicious breading. It's true. You can eat it without stirring up a high-carb storm. This recipe calls for chicken breasts, but you can use any chicken parts you like and you may leave the skin on if you desire. Serve with a side of Mock Mashed Potatoes (page 218) and Magic Rolls (page 22) or Elegant Biscuits (page 28) from Chapter 2.

PREPARATION TIME: 45 minutes (including making gravy). TOTAL COOKING TIME: 50 minutes.

SERVING SIZE: ¼ total yield. AMOUNT PER SERVING: 6.5 grams of carb, 38.1 grams of protein. NUMBER OF SERVINGS: 4.

		CHO (g)	PRO (g)
4	boneless, skinless chicken breast halves	0	108.8
1	cup Bread Crumbs I (page 25)	10.8	22.8
2	eggs, lightly beaten	1.2	12.0
1	teaspoon poultry seasoning (optional)	0.8	0
	salt to taste	0	0
	freshly ground black pepper to taste	0	0
4	tablespoons coconut oil	0	0
PAN GRAVY*			
1	cup broth or stock (see page 80)	1.0	3.0
1	cup heavy or light cream	6.4	4.8
	salt to taste	0	0
	freshly ground black pepper to taste	0	0
1	tablespoon Wondra flour (optional)	5.8	0.8
	Total	*26.0*	*152.2*

Preheat oven to 250°F.

Wash chicken and pat dry with paper towels. (*Optional:* For the tastiest, juiciest chicken, wash the night before, and when still wet, sprinkle liberally with Kosher or coarse salt, cover tightly, and refrigerate overnight. Rinse well and pat dry, then proceed with the recipe below.)

Put bread crumbs in a bowl large enough to hold individual chicken pieces. Mix with poultry seasoning, salt, and pepper. Put beaten eggs in another bowl.

---

* If you like, you can thicken the sauce slightly and save reducing time with 1 tablespoon of Wondra flour. This adds about 1.5 grams of carb per serving. Add the flour when you pour the broth in the skillet before it starts to simmer. Sprinkle flour over the top and whisk until smooth.

Dip chicken pieces first in the beaten egg, then coat well with bread crumbs. Place on a platter.

Heat a large, heavy skillet over medium-low heat. Heat coconut oil. Add the chicken pieces. Cook very slowly for about 20 minutes on each side or until done. How long this takes depends on the thickness of the pieces; chicken must be well done but will get tough if overcooked. You can check doneness with an instant meat thermometer; it should read 165°F. Low-carb bread crumbs tend to darken more quickly than ordinary bread crumbs. To keep them a light golden color, check often and turn heat to a lower setting if needed. Add more oil if needed. When the chicken is done, put the pieces on an ovenproof platter and keep warm in the oven. Keep the skillet hot.

To make the gravy, add broth to the hot skillet and scrape up loose particles. Simmer for about 5 to 10 minutes or until the liquid is reduced to about two-thirds of original amount. Add the cream. Simmer on low until the sauce is reduced further and has the desired thickness. (The gravy will continue to thicken a bit once removed from the direct heat.) Season with salt and pepper. When ready to serve, pour the gravy in a gravy boat.

Sweet-and-Sour Chicken

Another all-time favorite. This chicken must bake in the Sweet-and-Sour Sauce (below) for about an hour. (The meal tastes even better the next day—it is well worth making ahead if you expect company or are having an especially busy day.) The recipe calls for chicken breasts. You can use any combination of chicken pieces and cook them with the skin on or off, as you like. Serve with pasta. Check out pasta recipes in Chapter 6. Otherwise, have Magic Rolls handy (page 22).

PREPARATION TIME: 30 minutes. BAKING TIME: 1 hour.
SERVING SIZE: ¼ total yield. AMOUNT PER SERVING: 8.6 grams of carb, 31.0 grams of protein. NUMBER OF SERVINGS: 4 to 5

		CHO (g)	PRO (g)
4	boneless, skinless chicken breast halves	0	108.8
2	tablespoons coconut oil	0	0
	salt to taste	0	0
	freshly ground black pepper to taste	0	0
SWEET-AND-SOUR SAUCE			
½	cup drained and rinsed black soybeans	3.2	6.9
2	tablespoons butter	0	0
¾	cup finely chopped onion	8.3	1.3
1	cup canned, crushed tomatoes	12.0	4.0
1	cup stock or broth (page 80)	1.0	3.0
1	cup dry white wine	1.6	0.0
1	teaspoon hickory smoke liquid	3.0	0.0
½	teaspoon garlic powder	1.2	0.0
	salt to taste	0	0
	freshly ground black pepper to taste	0	0
4	packets Splenda sugar substitute (or to taste)	4.0	0
	Total (with sauce)	*34.3*	*124.0*

Preheat oven to 325°F. Butter or oil a medium-size ovenproof casserole dish.

Mash soybeans in a food processor or blender.

To make the sauce, heat a small skillet over medium heat. Add butter. When butter foams, sauté onion lightly. Put onion and all other sauce ingredients in a 2-quart saucepan. Simmer sauce gently for about 10 to 15 minutes while you prepare and brown the chicken pieces.

Wash chicken, and pat dry with paper towels. Cut each breast in bite-size pieces. Heat a large, heavy skillet over medium heat. Add coconut oil. Add chicken to the hot oil and brown quickly on both sides (for about 1 minute). Sprinkle the chicken with salt and pepper. Transfer chicken pieces to the casserole dish.

Pour the sauce over the chicken. Dot with butter. Bake, uncovered, for about 1 hour. Serve immediately.

Variation: Meatballs in Sweet-and-Sour Sauce
(Swedish Meatballs)

This is another way to please low carbers. It makes for a piquant dish; the meatballs are delicious when simmered in this sauce. Prepare one recipe of Super Meatballs (page 132). Make the meatballs small, about ¾ inch in diameter. They need less cooking time than larger meatballs. Because the sauce will simmer for about only half the time with the meat, give it a little headstart, simmering for about 30 minutes while you brown the meatballs in a large, heavy skillet. When they are browned, add the sauce and simmer the meatballs in it for about 20 to 25 minutes or until done. Season to taste. This recipe serves four but can easily be multiplied. You can make it a day ahead. You can also freeze this dish. A serving, including about ½ cup sauce, has 12.3 grams of carb and 33.2 grams of protein.

Cheesy Broccoli Chicken

This cheesy one-dish chicken meal is complete enough to serve with just a dinner salad in any season or coupled with slices of a fresh, ripe tomato in the summer when they're at their best. This delight is best served bubbling right from the oven, but if needed, you can make it ahead. Cover the baking dish tightly and refrigerate as soon as it is cool enough. Reheat it at 350°F until bubbly and hot, then take it as a covered dish to a potluck supper. Double or even triple the recipe for bigger gatherings.

PREPARATION TIME: 40 to 45 minutes. BROILING TIME: 3 to 5 minutes.
SERVING SIZE: ⅙ total yield. AMOUNT PER SERVING: 8.9 grams of carb, 43.6 grams of protein. NUMBER OF SERVINGS: 6

		CHO (g)	PRO (g)
6	boneless, skinless chicken breast halves	0	163.2
1	large bunch broccoli, cut into florets (about 1 pound)	9.6	14.4
5	tablespoons unsalted butter	0	0
3	tablespoons olive oil	0	0
1	pound large white mushrooms, cleaned and sliced	16.0	8.0
2	tablespoons lemon pepper	5.0	0
2	tablespoons unbleached, all-purpose white flour	11.5	1.6
½	cup chicken stock	0.5	1.5
½	cup dry white wine	0.8	0
1¾	cups shredded Swiss cheese	7.0	56.7
1	teaspoon salt	0	0
1	teaspoon white pepper	1.0	0
½	cup Jarlsberg cheese (regular Swiss is fine, too)	2.0	16.2
	Total	*53.4*	*261.6*

Butter an ovenproof baking dish large enough to hold the chicken and vegetables.

Wash chicken and pat dry with paper towels. (*Optional:* For the tastiest, juiciest chicken, wash the night before, and while still wet, sprinkle liberally with Kosher or coarse salt, cover tightly, and refrigerate overnight. Rinse well and pat dry, then proceed with the recipe below.)

Steam broccoli florets until al dente, about 3 to 6 minutes. Set aside.

Melt 1 tablespoon of the butter with the olive oil in a large, heavy skillet over low heat. Place the chicken pieces in the skillet in a single layer. Increase the heat to medium-high and cook until juices run clear when you prick the chicken with a fork, about 3 to 5 minutes on each side. Remove chicken to a heat-safe platter and set aside.

Preheat broiler to high setting.

Melt another 2 tablespoons of the butter in the skillet in which you just cooked the chicken. Add the mushroom slices and cook over medium-high heat until tender, about 3 to 5 minutes.

Arrange the cooked broccoli in the bottom of the buttered baking dish.

Season chicken breasts with lemon pepper and arrange atop the broccoli in the baking dish.

Melt the remaining 2 tablespoons of butter in a 1-quart saucepan over low heat. Whisk in the flour and cook, stirring constantly, about 3 minutes. Pour the chicken stock and wine into the butter–flour mixture, whisking constantly until thoroughly blended. Continue to cook, stirring constantly, until sauce thickens and coats the back of a spoon.

Add the shredded Swiss cheese to the sauce, stirring until melted. Season with salt and pepper as directed (or to taste).

Pour the sauce over the chicken and broccoli. Arrange mushroom slices on top. Sprinkle with the shredded Jarlsberg cheese. Broil, about 6 inches from heat, until the top is bubbly and golden, about 3 to 5 minutes. Watch very carefully to prevent burning the cheese on top.

Blackened Chicken

If you love spicy foods, you won't be able to resist the Cajun flavor of these roasted chicken breasts. This dish is so easy to fix, you'll find yourself making it again and again. If you do, mix up the blackening spices in larger quantities and store them in an airtight container for an even easier dish the next time. The recipe can be multiplied easily. Pair these spicy treats with Baked Black Soybeans (page 212) and Coleslaw Supreme (page 90) for an easy alfresco summer dinner.

PREPARATION TIME: 15 minutes. BAKING TIME: 20 to 30 minutes.
SERVING SIZE: 1 breast. AMOUNT PER SERVING: 1.6 grams of carb, 30.8 grams of protein. NUMBER OF SERVINGS: 4.

	CHO (g)	PRO (g)
4 boneless chicken breast halves, with skin	0	120.8
1 tablespoon olive oil	0	0
BLACKENING MIXTURE		
1 tablespoon paprika	1.8	0.9
2 teaspoons dried oregano	0.8	0
2 teaspoons garlic salt	1.0	0
1 teaspoon cayenne pepper	0.5	1.0
2 teaspoons freshly ground black pepper	2.0	0.6
Total	*6.1*	*123.3*

Preheat the oven to 425°F. Make the blackening mixture by combining all the spices in an airtight bag. Then pour the spice mixture on a plate and set aside.

Wash chicken and pat dry with paper towels. (*Optional:* For the tastiest, juiciest chicken, wash the night before, and while still wet, sprinkle liberally with Kosher or coarse salt, cover tightly, and refrigerate overnight. Rinse well and pat dry, then proceed with the recipe below.)

Rub each chicken breast in a little olive oil. Roll each chicken breast in the spice mixture, coating evenly.

Place breasts in a single layer in a 9- by 13-inch baking pan. (If making more, be sure your pan holds all the chicken in a single layer—or use a larger pan or more than one.)

Bake the chicken until done, about 20 to 30 minutes. The cayenne and paprika will make it difficult to see a "clear" juice when you pierce the breasts, so be sure to use an instant-read meat thermometer to check for doneness. For chicken it should read 165°F when inserted into the thickest part of the meat.

Island Wings

A great treat for a casual family dinner, with enough left over to pack in a lunchbox the next day. Perfect for picnics, it's an easy way to feed a party crowd.

PREPARATION TIME: 25 minutes. GRILLING TIME: depends on size of grill, 7 to 10 minutes per batch.

SERVING SIZE: $1/10$ total yield. AMOUNT PER SERVING: 2.8 grams of carb, 45.9 grams of protein. NUMBER OF SERVINGS: 10.

		CHO (g)	PRO (g)
10	pounds chicken wings	0	449.0
1	cup fresh lime juice	20.8	1.6
½	cup dark rum	0	0
¼	cup soy sauce	4.0	8.0
4	jalapeño peppers, thinly sliced	3.4	0.5
	Total	*28.2*	*459.1*

The night before you intend to cook the wings, you'll need to marinate them to get that delicious island flavor. Using a sharp knife, cleaver, or poultry shears, separate the wings at the joint, making a "wing" and a "drumette." Wash and pat all pieces dry with paper towels.

Mix together lime juice, rum, soy sauce, and peppers. Place chicken pieces in a nonmetal container and pour the lime juice mixture over them. Add enough water so that all chicken is covered. Cover container and refrigerate overnight

Preheat grill on medium-high or prepare a bed of hot coals in the grill. Remove wings from refrigerator and drain well. Grill wings over hot coals until done, about 7 to 10 minutes, turning often to prevent burning.

Variation: Broiled Island Wings

When it's not grilling season, you can broil the wings on high or in a preheated 500°F oven about 6 inches from the heat. Cook about 4 minutes on each side.

Parmesan Chicken Sauté

An inexpensive and delightfully crisp rendition of panfried chicken cutlets, these breasts make an easy but elegant entree for the family or for company. Pair them with a sauté of baby winter squashes when it's cold out or with springtime vegetables in the warm months. Either way, you'll love the chicken's delicate crisp outside and juicy, tender meat. Bigger appetites might want a double serving! And for little ones, you might use a sharp metal cookie cutter to shape the flattened chicken breast into stars or favorite animal shapes before sautéing.

PREPARATION TIME: 20 minutes. COOKING TIME: 1 hour (unless all the chicken is cooked at the same time).

SERVING SIZE: 1 breast. AMOUNT PER SERVING: 1.0 gram of carb, 37.1 grams of protein. NUMBER OF SERVINGS: 6.

		CHO (g)	PRO (g)
6	boneless, skinless chicken breast halves	0	163.2
2	eggs, slightly beaten	1.2	12.0
1	teaspoon salt	1.0	0
1	teaspoon pepper	0	0
1	cup grated Parmesan cheese	4.0	47.6
3	tablespoons olive oil or coconut oil (or as needed)	0	0
	Total	6.2	222.8

Wash and pat the chicken breasts dry with paper towels. Pound them to flatten, using a rolling pin or the flat side of a meat mallet. (This is less messy if you put single pieces in tie-type plastic bags to pound, but do not tie.)

Use bowls large enough to hold the chicken pieces. Have the beaten eggs ready in one bowl and the Parmesan cheese in another.

Dip each chicken breast in the beaten egg; coat evenly. Sprinkle with salt and pepper, then roll in the Parmesan cheese.

Preheat a large, heavy skillet. Add the olive or coconut oil. Put coated chicken in the heated oil and sauté slowly, turning to brown and cook evenly on both sides. Keep temperature on the low side; the Parmesan cheese tends to burn fairly easily. (Cook half the chicken at one time and keep warm in the oven preheated to 300°F or use two skillets large enough to cook all of the chicken at the same time.) Do not crowd breasts. Add more oil during cooking, if needed. To get a delicious, crisp chicken that is fully cooked, slow and easy is the trick here. (You can always use an instant-read meat thermometer to check for doneness—insert from the side; chicken should register 165°F when inserted into the thickest part of the meat.)

Rich Sour Cream Chicken

Busy cooks will appreciate the ease with which this recipe goes together. Pop it in the oven and you have an hour to toss a salad or sauté some veggies to round out a filling dinner. The creamy sauce is perfect over Mock Mashed Potatoes (page 218), superb over Supreme Pasta (page 172), or even to sop up with Magic Rolls (page 22). This recipe is easy to adapt to larger or smaller portions.

PREPARATION TIME: 15 minutes. BAKING TIME: 1 hour.
SERVING SIZE: 1 breast. AMOUNT PER SERVING: 1.7 grams of carb, 43.1 grams of protein. NUMBER OF SERVINGS: 8.

		CHO (g)	PRO (g)
8	chicken breast halves with skin and bones	0	322.7
1½	cups crushed pork rinds (about 20 rinds)	0	12.2
1½	cups sour cream	12.0	9.6
1½	teaspoons salt	0	0
1	teaspoon dried thyme	0.6	0
1	teaspoon paprika	0.6	0
1	teaspoon garlic salt	0.5	0.6
	Total	*13.7*	*345.1*

Preheat oven to 350°F. Butter or oil an ovenproof baking dish (or broiler pan) large enough to hold the chicken.

Wash the chicken and pat dry with paper towels. (Optional: For the tastiest, juiciest chicken, wash the night before, and while still wet, sprinkle liberally with Kosher or coarse salt, cover tightly, and refrigerate overnight. Rinse well and pat dry, then proceed with the recipe below, reducing the salt to ¾ teaspoon in the sauce.)

Place the crushed pork rinds on a plate or a piece of waxed paper. In a wide, shallow bowl, mix together the sour cream, salt, thyme, paprika, and garlic salt. Dip the chicken into the sour cream mixture, then roll it in the crushed pork rinds.

Place the chicken pieces in the baking dish or pan. Bake for 1 hour or until tender. (Check for doneness with an instant-read meat thermometer inserted in the thickest part of the meat. Chicken should register 165°F when done.)

Variation: Crumby Sour Cream Chicken

You can substitute ¾ cup Bread Crumbs I or II (pages 25 and 26) for the pork rinds. Mix crumbs with 1 tablespoon grated Parmesan cheese and add small amounts of salt and freshly ground pepper. It will add 1.0 gram of carb per serving and 2.3 grams of protein.

Barbecued Peanut Butter Chicken

This chicken is a marvelous treat. It's basted with a spicy peanut butter–vinegar sauce as it cooks over the coals.

PREPARATION TIME: 15 minutes. GRILLING TIME: 1½ hours.
SERVING SIZE: ½ broiler. AMOUNT PER SERVING: 2.3 grams of carb, about 41.0 grams of protein. NUMBER OF SERVINGS: 6.

	CHO (g)	PRO (g)
3 chicken broilers (under 2 pounds each), split	0	240.0
salt to taste	0	0
freshly ground black pepper to taste	0	0
2 tablespoons peanut oil (or as needed)	0	0
BARBECUE SAUCE		
1 cup plus 2 tablespoons white wine vinegar	0	0
6 tablespoons lemon juice	7.8	0
1 tablespoon peanut oil	0	0
1 tablespoon butter	0	0
2 teaspoons chili powder (or as desired)	1.0	0.6
1 tablespoon smooth peanut butter	2.2	4.5
1 teaspoon flaked celery seed	0.6	0
salt to taste (about 2 teaspoons)	0	0
freshly ground black pepper to taste (about 2 teaspoons)	2.0	0.6
Total	*13.4*	*245.7*

Preheat grill or start fire in the grill.

Thoroughly wash broilers and pat dry with paper towels. Rub the chicken pieces with peanut oil, salt, and pepper. Set aside.

To make the barbecue sauce, combine all the sauce ingredients in a 1-quart saucepan. Mix well and heat through (make sure the peanut butter is melted). Set aside.

When the grill is ready, put the chicken pieces on it. Baste them with the sauce as they cook; turn chicken often. Grill for about 1½ hours or until completely done, but chicken should register 165°F when done.

Variation: Broiled Peanut Butter Chicken

Rainy day? Just move the cooking indoors. Preheat the oven at 400°F. Put the split broilers on a greased rack, skin side up. Cook for about 5 minutes, then baste lightly with the peanut sauce. Bake for a total of about 30 minutes, basting repeatedly. Turn chicken and continue basting. If you run out of sauce, scoop some from the bottom of the broiling pan. Bake an additional 30 minutes or until chicken is done. Test with an instead-read meat thermometer inserted into the thickest part of the meat. Chicken should register 165°F when done.

Sesame Thighs

Savory and full of good-quality fats, this recipe will become a family favorite. Pair it with Mock Mashed Potatoes (page 218) and a dinner salad for some low-carb comfort. Easy to make in large batches.

PREPARATION TIME: 15 minutes. BAKING TIME: 45 minutes.
SERVING SIZE: 2 thighs. AMOUNT PER SERVING: 1.0 gram of carb, 34.7 grams
   of protein. NUMBER OF SERVINGS: 3.

		CHO (g)	PRO (g)
6	skinless chicken thighs	0	97.4
1	tablespoon butter	0	0
1½	tablespoons soy sauce	1.5	3.0
2	tablespoons sesame seeds	1.6	3.6
	freshly ground pepper to taste	0	0
	Total	*3.1*	*104.0*

Wash chicken and pat dry with paper towels. (*Optional:* For the tastiest, juiciest chicken, wash the night before, and while still wet, sprinkle liberally with Kosher or coarse salt, cover tightly, and refrigerate overnight. Rinse well and pat dry, then proceed with the recipe below.)

In a bowl large enough to hold the chicken, mix soy sauce and pepper. Coat each breast with the soy mixture. Pour any remaining mixture over the chicken, cover, and refrigerate for at least 30 minutes.

Preheat oven to 375°F. Prepare a shallow baking dish with butter in it, put dish in oven, and let butter melt while oven is preheating. Remove baking dish from oven when the butter is melted. Roll each chicken thigh in the butter, coating on all sides, and arrange in a single layer in the dish. Sprinkle sesame seeds on top of each piece of chicken.

Return baking dish to the oven and bake for 45 minutes, turning the thighs two or three times during the cooking process to ensure even cooking all the way through (chicken is fully cooked when temperature registers 165°F).

Baked Chicken Salad Casserole

This baked salad is really an easy chicken casserole for the family or a great budget saver as a party entree. Your guests will rave about it and demand the recipe. You can assemble it several hours ahead of time, cover tightly, refrigerate, then pop it in the oven a half hour or so before the guests arrive. Toss a big garden salad, put some Garlic Bread (page 26) in a basket, and bring out a fabulous Scrumptious Low-Carb Cheesecake (page 269) for dessert (which took just 20 minutes to make the day before). Sit back and enjoy your own party!

PREPARATION TIME: 15 minutes. BAKING TIME: 25 minutes.
SERVING SIZE: ⅛ total yield. AMOUNT PER SERVING: 2.8 grams of carb, 28.8 grams of protein. NUMBER OF SERVINGS: 8.

	CHO (g)	PRO (g)
4 cups cooked, bite-size pieces of skinless chicken	0	172.0
4 cups diced celery	4.8	2.0
2 teaspoons salt	0	0
½ teaspoon dried tarragon	0.7	0
¼ cup chopped scallions (green and white parts)	1.2	0
1 tablespoon lemon juice	1.3	0
2 cups Basic Mayonnaise (page 239)	0	0
¼ cup extra-dry vermouth	0	0
¾ cup toasted sliced almonds	9.0	18.0
¾ cup plain, crushed pork rinds (about 12)	0	7.4
¼ cup sesame seeds (not toasted)	3.0	7.0
½ cup grated Parmesan cheese	2.0	23.8
Total	*22.0*	*230.2*

In a large bowl, mix the chicken pieces, celery, salt, tarragon, scallion, lemon juice, mayonnaise, vermouth, and almonds. Taste at this point for seasonings; add salt if necessary. Cover tightly and refrigerate for at least 1 hour. (You may refrigerate for several hours at this point and bake the dish later—for example, put it together in the morning and bake when you get home from work.)

Preheat oven to 350°F when you are ready to bake. Lightly butter or oil a shallow baking dish.

Spoon the chicken salad into the baking dish and top with the crushed pork rinds, sesame seeds, and Parmesan cheese. Bake until completely heated through and the cheese melts and just begins to brown slightly, approximately 25 minutes.

Variation: Crumby Chicken Salad Casserole

You can substitute ¾ cup Bread Crumbs I or II (pages 25 and 26) for the pork rinds. Mix crumbs with 1 tablespoon grated Parmesan cheese and add small amounts of salt and freshly ground black pepper. It will add 1.0 gram of carb per serving and 2.3 grams of protein.

Easy Turkey Casserole

What to do with the left over turkey? Here's a recipe that is so good you might not want to wait for the traditional turkey-eating season. If that's the case, just poach a fresh turkey breast in chicken stock, let it cool, dice it, and you're good to go. The recipe can be multiplied easily for potlucks, family reunions, or any time you need to feed a big crowd on a budget.

PREPARATION TIME: 20 minutes. COOKING TIME: 25 to 30 minutes.
SERVING SIZE: ¼ total yield. AMOUNT PER SERVING: 3.9 grams of carb, 32.9 grams of protein. NUMBER OF SERVINGS: 4.

		CHO (g)	PRO (g)
2	cups cooked, bite-size pieces of turkey	0	84.8
2	cups diced celery	4.8	2.0
5	tablespoons minced scallions (green and white parts)	1.3	0
1	cup Basic Mayonnaise (page 239)	0	0
1	tablespoon lemon juice	1.3	0
¼	cup canned chopped pimiento	1.5	0.5
½	cup sliced almonds	6.0	12.0
1	cup grated Monterey Jack cheese	0.8	28.0
½	cup plain, crushed pork rinds (about 8)	0	4.9
	Total	*15.7*	*131.2*

In a large bowl, mix together the turkey pieces, celery, scallion, mayonnaise, lemon juice, and pimiento. (You may cover tightly and refrigerate for several hours at this point and bake the dish later—for example, put it together in the morning and bake when you get home from work.)

Mix together the almonds, grated cheese, and pork rinds. Set aside.

Preheat oven to 350°F when you are ready to bake. Oil or butter a 2-quart casserole dish.

Spoon the turkey mixture into the casserole dish and sprinkle the cheese mixture evenly on top. Bake until completely heated through and the cheese melts and just begins to brown slightly, approximately 25 to 30 minutes.

Variation: Crumby Turkey Casserole

If you like, you can substitute ¼ cup Bread Crumbs I or II (pages 25 and 26) for the pork rinds. Mix crumbs with 1 tablespoon grated Parmesan cheese and add small amounts of salt and freshly ground black pepper. It will add 0.7 grams of carb per serving and 20 grams of protein.

Turkey Loaf

You can make this from leftover turkey. It's a scrumptious meal that you can throw together in a food processor and pop in the oven. You can make the same dish with leftover chicken. Yum!

PREPARATION TIME: 15 minutes. BAKING TIME: 35 to 45 minutes.

SERVING SIZE: ¼ total yield. AMOUNT PER SERVING: 4.6 grams of carb, 32.4 grams of protein. NUMBER OF SERVINGS: 4.

		CHO (g)	PRO (g)
½	cup Bread Crumbs I (page 25)	5.4	11.4
⅓	cup light cream	2.2	1.6
12	ounces skinless cooked turkey (dark and white meat), cut into chunks	0	99.0
1	medium onion, quartered	5.5	0.9
10	large, black, canned olives	1.0	0
2	tablespoons drained and rinsed capers	2.0	0
2	tablespoons freshly chopped parsley (or 1 tablespoon dried)	0	0
2	ounces Canadian-style bacon, coarsely chopped	0.8	13.8
½	teaspoon garlic powder	1.2	0
	salt to taste (about ¾ teaspoon)	0	0
	freshly ground black pepper to taste	0.0	0.0
1	egg yolk	0.3	2.8
	Total	*18.4*	*129.5*

Preheat oven to 350°F. If you make a hand-shaped loaf (recommended), use a small jelly roll pan (with an outer edge). Otherwise, use a 4- by 8-inch loaf pan. Whichever you choose, butter or oil it lightly.

In a small bowl, combine bread crumbs with the cream; stir and set aside.

Put all ingredients except the bread crumb–cream mixture and the egg yolk in the bowl of a food processor. Pulse briefly and check often. You want to retain some coarseness (and avoid mush). Taste and adjust seasoning. Finally, add the bread crumb–cream mixture and the egg yolk. Pulse once more. (You can do all of this by hand, too. However, if you do it that way, chop all ingredients finely before you mash them together with a fork or a potato masher.)

Shape the mixture into a freestanding loaf or fit it in the loaf pan. Dot with butter. Bake, uncovered, for 35 to 45 minutes or until lightly browned. Cool for about ½ hour before slicing (it makes slicing easier).

Serve with a drizzle of hot Cranberry Sauce (page 299). The sauce, if prepared according to instructions, has 1.9 grams of carb per serving. You can heat it in the microwave.

Baked Apple Onion Stuffing

This baked stuffing will not only make the traditional turkey dinner more wonderful, but it can also do double duty as a side dish. A regular stuffing averages 23.0 grams of carb in ½ cup; this one has 7.8 grams. Prepare the croutons used in the stuffing ahead of time if you like. You can even freeze them. use Croutons I (page 24) or gluten-free Croutons II (page 25).

PREPARATION TIME: 30 minutes. BAKING TIME: 35 to 40 minutes.

SERVING SIZE: ⅛ of recipe. AMOUNT PER SERVING: 7.8 grams of carb, 7.0 grams of protein. NUMBER OF SERVINGS: 8.

		CHO (g)	PRO (g)
1	Recipe Herbed Croutons I (page 24)	14.4	28.5
2	cups peeled, chopped apples	28.0	0
1	tablespoon lemon juice	1.3	0
1	cup finely chopped onion	11.0	1.8
½	cup finely chopped celery	1.2	0
3	tablespoons olive oil or coconut oil	0	0
2	tablespoons butter	0	0
	salt to taste (about ½ teaspoon)	0	0
	freshly ground black pepper to taste	0	0
½	teaspoon garlic powder	1.2	0
½	cup chicken broth or stock (see page 80)	0.5	1.5
½	cup light or heavy cream	3.2	2.4
3	egg yolks	0.9	8.4
2	tablespoons chopped fresh parsley (or 1 tablespoon dried parsley)	0	0
2	tablespoons butter (optional)	0	0
¼	cup grated Parmesan or Romano cheese	1.0	11.9
	Total	62.7	54.5

Preheat oven to 325°F. Butter or oil a medium ovenproof casserole dish or heavy-gauge metal baking pan.

Put the croutons in a large mixing bowl. In a separate bowl, drizzle lemon juice over the chopped apples. Set aside. Chop onion and celery.

Heat a large, heavy skillet over medium-low heat. Add oil and butter. Sauté the onion until it becomes translucent. Add celery and apples. Cook over low heat until apples are tender. If skillet gets too dry, add a few tablespoons of broth. Stir in salt, pepper, and garlic powder. Add this mix to the croutons and stir thoroughly. Transfer all to the baking dish.

In a small bowl beat egg yolks until smooth. Beat in cream and broth. Pour the liquid over the crouton mixture and stir it in lightly with a fork. Sprinkle with the Parmesan cheese and dot with butter. Bake uncovered for about 30 to 35 minutes or until the dressing is lightly browned on top. Sprinkle with parsley and serve.

You can also prepare the stuffing a few hours or even a day ahead of time. Just leave off the liquid and refrigerate the casserole. Add liquid when you are ready to bake. Increase baking time by a few minutes.

Variation: Baked Mushroom Stuffing

This is another irresistible stuffing where mushrooms provide the main flavor—not just one but three different kinds. Follow the directions for Baked Apple-Onion Dressing but reduce onion to ½ cup and omit celery and apples. Replace these ingredients with 12 ounces mushrooms. Choose portabella, shiitake, and white mushrooms or other combinations (you can also get by with just one or two kinds, if you like). Add 10 large, canned, black olives, chopped, or 5 fresh olives in brine, such as Kalamata, pitted and chopped. Wipe mushrooms clean with a damp paper towel; remove tough parts of stems and slice in ½-inch pieces. Sauté the onion for 1 minute and add the mushrooms (add some butter and oil if needed). Cook mushrooms until tender, about 5 minutes. Add olives and stir for another minute. Combine with croutons, season, and put in the casserole dish. Finish as directed. A serving of this stuffing (based on 8) has 5.2 grams of carb; protein remains virtually unchanged.

Variation: Baked Celery Stuffing

A great stuffing, probably unlike any you have tasted before. Celery gives it a lively and interesting flavor. Follow the directions for Baked Apple Onion Stuffing on page 128, but reduce onion to ½ cup and omit apples. Increase celery to 2 cups. Add 10 fresh, chopped, pitted olives in brine, such as Kalamata, or 15 large, canned, black olives, chopped, and 3 tablespoons drained and mashed capers. Also add 1 teaspoon dried sage and 1 teaspoon dried thyme. Add olives, capers, sage, and thyme after the celery has cooked for about 2 minutes. Combine all with croutons, season, and put in the casserole dish. Finish as directed. A serving of this stuffing (based on 6) has 4.9 grams of carb; protein remains virtually unchanged.

Stuffed Blue Cheese Patties

Tasty, savory, and oh so easy, these patties offer a new twist on the traditional cheeseburger. Those who want to turn up the heat a bit can even add a tablespoon of hot roasted green chile to their burger for an additional 1 gram of carb. You can serve them naked with a salad or with our low-carb Magic Rolls (burger size, page 22), or the old-fashioned way, with lettuce, tomato, and plenty of mustard (don't forget to count those carbs, too).

PREPARATION TIME: 10–15 minutes. COOKING TIME: 8 to 12 minutes.

SERVING SIZE: 1 patty. AMOUNT PER SERVING: 1.7 grams of carb, 43.2 grams of protein. NUMBER OF SERVINGS: 4.

		CHO (g)	PRO (g)
2	pounds lean ground beef	0	160.0
½	cup crumbled blue cheese	2.0	12.0
2	tablespoons sour cream	1.0	0.8
¼	cup Basic Mayonnaise (page 239)	0	0
¼	cup finely chopped red onion	2.8	0
1	teaspoon salt	1.0	0
1	teaspoon pepper	0	0
	Total	*6.8*	*172.8*

Divide the beef into eight equal portions on a sheet of waxed paper or aluminum foil. Press each portion into a patty about ¼ inch thick.

Mix all the other ingredients together and divide the mixture equally between four of the patties, placing it in the center of each patty, leaving some space around the outer edge to seal the patties. Put one of the remaining four patties on top of those with the blue cheese stuffing. Press or pinch the edges of the patties to seal firmly.

Lightly grease a skillet or griddle with a bit of coconut oil, and, when hot, place the patties on it. Cook for approximately 4 to 6 minutes on each side or until cooked through, without residual pink color. Ground beef is safest cooked through to at least medium or medium-well. Check with an instant-read meat thermometer if in doubt.

Variation: Grilled Blue Cheese Patties

This recipe works well in clamshell-type home grills, such as the George Foreman Grill, or on an outdoor grill. Cook about 8 minutes in a preheated clamshell-type grill or about 5 minutes per side on a medium-hot outdoor grill. Check to be sure no pink color remains in the meat.

Best Meat Loaf

Everyone has a favorite meat loaf recipe. This one evolved over time and has become a favorite in our homes. It has simple ingredients, is quick and easy to make, and it is light and moist. Use Bread Crumbs I (page 25) or gluten-free Bread Crumbs II (page 26) from Chapter 2. For an elegant appearance (and easy slicing) you may want to shape the meat like a loaf of bread. For the best-tasting ground beef, select a fairly large chunk of chuck or sirloin yourself and have the butcher remove the gristle, grind the meat for you, and package it in sizes you normally use. Or grind the meat yourself. If you prefer, use a combination of beef, veal, and pork or any two. Leftover meat loaf tastes great as sandwiches on Magic Rolls (page 22) or any kind of bread.

PREPARATION TIME: 15 minutes. BAKING TIME: 1 hour.
SERVING SIZE: ¼ loaf (2 thick slices). AMOUNT PER SERVING: 4.1 grams of
  carb, 32.6 grams of protein. NUMBER OF SERVINGS: 4 to 5.

	CHO (g)	PRO (g)
⅔ cup heavy cream	4.2	3.2
½ cup Bread Crumbs I (page 25)	5.4	11.4
1¼ to 1¾ pounds lean ground beef:		
chuck or top sirloin	0	100.0
3 tablespoons freshly minced parsley		
(or 1 tablespoon dried)	0	0
½ cup finely minced onion	5.5	0.9
salt to taste (about 1 teaspoon)	0	0
freshly ground black pepper to taste	0	0
1 ounce Parmesan cheese	1.0	11.9
1 egg yolk	0.3	2.8
Total	*16.4*	*130.2*

Preheat oven to 325°F. Put a 12- by 14-piece of aluminum foil on a cookie sheet or jelly roll pan or lightly grease a 4- by 8-inch baking pan.

Put cream and bread crumbs in the bowl of a food processor or mixer or put them in a medium mixing bowl. Stir lightly and soak for about 5 minutes.

Add ground beef, parsley, onion, salt, pepper, Parmesan cheese, and egg yolk in the bowl with the soaking bread crumbs. Process just until lightly mixed (it is important not to overmix) or do this by hand. Place on top of the aluminum foil and shape into a loaf about 12 or 13 inches long. Lightly build up a slight edge with the aluminum foil (unless you are using a jelly roll pan or a regular baking pan). Bake for about 1 hour or until done. Ground beef is safest cooked through to at least medium or medium-well. Check with an instant-read meat thermometer if in doubt. Wait for about 15 minutes to slice.

Variation: Sizzling Meat Loaf Steaks

These steaks are easy to make, taste fabulous, and don't cost much. Follow the directions for making Best Meat Loaf on page 131. Shape the meat loaf into a rectangle or so that it fits into a 4- by 8-inch baking pan. Bake it for about 40 minutes. (It will not be done.) Put the loaf in the fridge until you want to make the steaks—a few hours or not longer than overnight. When you are ready to cook the steaks, slice the meat loaf in four. Heat a large, heavy skillet over medium-high heat. Add 1 or 2 tablespoons coconut oil. Brown the slices quickly on both sides. Reduce heat and cook the slices for about 15 minutes, turning them once. Check for doneness with an instant-read meat thermometer. You can serve the steaks on a bed of Mock Mashed Potatoes (page 218) and drizzle with Cranberry Sauce (page 299). Amount per serving for steaks only is 4.1 grams of carb and 32.6 grams of protein.

Variation: Super Meatballs

Who does not like meatballs? These meatballs are easy to make and exceptionally tasty. Just follow the recipe for Best Meat Loaf on page 131, but shape the mixture into balls instead of a loaf. The recipe serves four and makes about twelve 1¾-inch meatballs or sixteen 1½-inch meatballs, but make any size you want. Carb and protein counts are the same as for the meat loaf. Cooking times are for large meatballs, so adjust accordingly.

The meatballs are delicious served plain, perhaps with a side of Mock Mashed Potatoes (page 218) and a steamed, buttered dish of asparagus with Jiffy Hollandaise Sauce (page 248). They take on a new dimension and can be turned into several different entrees if you allow them to simmer to perfection in a variety of marvelous sauces, such as Mock Marinara Sauce (page 134), Caper Sauce (page 136), or Barbecue Sauce (page 137). Serve over pasta; you have pasta recipes to choose from in Chapter 6. You can also quickly make tasty low-carb imitation pasta from crepes (page 45); you can serve this meal over waffles (page 53) or simply use Magic Rolls, either white or whole wheat (page 22). For a little extra work, you can have Best Garlic Bread (page 26). Country Rolls (page 37) go will with it, too. You'll find another sauce option—Sweet-and-Sour Sauce—on page 113.

Start out by browning the meatballs. Heat a heavy skillet over medium heat. Add about 2 tablespoons of coconut or olive oil to the hot skillet. Quickly brown the meatballs on all sides, taking care not to make them too dark. You may want to discard some of the accumulating fat. Reduce heat immediately. If you intend to cook meatballs without sauce, have ½ cup of broth on hand. Add small amounts of it to the pan, as needed, to keep it from getting dry. Sauté the meatballs for about 45 minutes or until done.

To cook the meatballs in a sauce, you have two choices: cook the sauce and meatballs in the skillet or cook them in the oven. Preheat oven to 300°F. Butter or oil a casserole dish and transfer the meatballs to it when they have been browned. Pour the sauce over the meatballs. Dot with a little butter (optional). Check after about 20 minutes. If the sauce has reduced quite a bit, cover the casserole for the remaining time. Aluminum foil is fine. If using a skillet, cover and occasionally stir the meatballs and sauce. Whichever method you use, cook the meatballs for about 45 to 60 minutes in the sauce. If you make very small meatballs, reduce this time.

Meatballs in Mock Marinara Sauce

Follow directions for making Best Meat Loaf on page 131 and Meatballs on page 132. Add 1 teaspoon each dried basil (0.7 gram of carb) and dried oregano (0.4 gram of carb) to the meat mixture. Make Mock Marinara Sauce (page 134) while the meatballs are browning or make it ahead of time. Add the sauce to the skillet with the meatballs (omit the broth) and simmer on very low for about 40 minutes or until meatballs are done. (Do not undercook ground beef.) Keep a lid on the skillet and stir occasionally. Remove lid for the last 10 or 15 minutes, especially if you want the sauce to thicken more. If you prefer, you can also preheat the oven to 325°F, butter an ovenproof casserole dish (with lid), add meatballs and sauce to it as soon as the meatballs have been browned, and bake for about 40 minutes or until the meatballs are done. For the meatballs only, based on a serving for four, there are 4.2 grams of carb and 31.8 grams of protein per serving. Serve with any pasta recipe from Chapter 6, including quick pasta made from crepes, and a zesty salad.

Mock Marinara Sauce

Use this sauce any time you need tomato sauce. Double or triple the recipe and freeze. It will come in handy.

PREPARATION TIME: 20 minutes. COOKING TIME: 1 to 1½ hours.
SERVING SIZE: ½ cup. AMOUNT PER SERVING (SAUCE ONLY): 5.1 grams of carb, 2.0 grams of protein. NUMBER OF SERVINGS: 6.

		CHO (g)	PRO (g)
2	tablespoons olive oil	0	0
2	tablespoons butter	0	0
¾	cup chopped onion	8.3	1.4
1	cup finely chopped celery	2.4	0
1½	cups stock or broth (page 80)	1.5	4.5
2	tablespoons tomato paste	5.0	2.0
1½	cups canned, crushed tomatoes	12.0	4.0
	salt to taste (1 teaspoon or more)	0	0
	freshly ground black pepper to taste	0	0
2	teaspoons dried basil	0.7	0
2	teaspoons dried oregano	0.8	0
	Total	*30.7*	*11.9*

Heat a medium-size heavy-bottomed saucepan over medium heat. Add the oil and butter. Add the onion when the butter foams (do not brown) and sauté for about 3 or 4 minutes. Add the celery and cook for an additional 3 minutes.

Add the broth and tomato paste to the saucepan. Whisk to dissolve paste. Add the remaining ingredients. Stir and simmer the sauce gently for about 15 minutes. For a smooth sauce, put it in a food processor or blender. If you are making the sauce only, without meatballs, cover and simmer for about 1½ hours, stirring occasionally. Add a little broth if the sauce gets too thick. Adjust seasoning.

Variation: Italian Meat Sauce

This is a rich meat sauce, easy to make, that you can use on many occasions. Simply follow directions for Mock Marinara Sauce. Use a larger saucepan. Let the sauce begin to simmer while you prepare the meat. Heat a medium-large, heavy skillet over medium-high heat. Add 2 to 3 tablespoons coconut oil to the hot skillet. Quickly brown 1¼ pounds lean ground beef (or a mixture of beef and uncooked Italian sausage) in the skillet, stirring as you do. Season with salt and freshly ground black pepper. When the meat has turned brown—it does not need to cook through—add it to the Mock Marinara Sauce.

Simmer the meat in the sauce for about 1½ to 2 hours. Keep heat very low. Adjust seasonings. The meat adds 120.0 grams of protein to the sauce. Makes 6 to 7 one-cup servings. A serving has 5.1 grams of carb and 22.0 grams of protein.

Variation: Slow-Cooked Sauce

You can cook any of these sauces—Meatballs in Mock Marinara Sauce, the Mock Marinara Sauce by itself, or the Italian Meat Sauce—in a slow cooker. Prepare all sauces to the point of simmering the night before. Store the sauce in the fridge and pour it in the slow cooker in the morning. Set the pot on low (or follow manufacturer's directions). You can cook the sauce all day and have it ready when you return. If the sauce is too thin, put it in a saucepan on the stovetop and simmer while you prepare the rest of dinner.

Meatballs in Caper Sauce

Follow directions for making Best Meat Loaf on page 131 and Meatballs on page 132. If you like capers, this meal is an out-of-this-world treat—good enough for company—yet you can make it quickly (and have it all cooked when your friends arrive). For directions to cook the meatballs in the sauce, see Meatballs in Marinara Sauce on page 133. For the Caper Sauce, see page 136. This sauce goes well with steamed, buttered cabbage and with pasta. Pasta recipes are in Chapter 6. Amount per serving, meatballs only (based on 4): 4.1 grams of carb, 31.8 grams of protein.

Caper Sauce

You are in for a treat when you cook meatballs in this sauce. But do not overlook it as a good sauce to serve over veggies, especially cabbage, and over fish.

PREPARATION TIME: 15 minutes. COOKING TIME: 1 hour.
SERVING SIZE: ½ cup. AMOUNT PER SERVING: 2.9 grams of carb, 4.3 grams of protein. NUMBER OF SERVINGS: 4.

		CHO (g)	PRO (g)
2½	cups broth or stock (page 80)	2.5	7.5
6	tablespoons butter (¾ stick)	0	0
2	tablespoons drained and rinsed capers	2.0	0
½	cup rinsed, drained and mashed black soybeans	3.2	6.9
1	teaspoon Dijon-style mustard	0.5	0.5
	salt to taste	0	0
	freshly ground black pepper to taste	0	0
½	cup cream	3.2	2.4
	Total	*11.4*	*17.3*

Put all the ingredients except for the cream in a medium saucepan and cook on medium-low heat. Turn down heat when the sauce bubbles and simmer for about 10 to 15 minutes before adding the sauce to the meatballs. If you bake the meatballs, add the cream to the sauce when you add it to the casserole. If you cook the meatballs in the skillet, add the cream last. Adjust the seasonings. This sauce freezes well.

Meatballs in Barbecue Sauce

Follow directions for making Best Meat Loaf on page 131 and Meat-
balls on page 132. If you like barbecue sauce, this meal is one you
will want to eat again and again. For directions to cook the meatballs
in the sauce, see Meatballs in Marinara Sauce on page 133. For the
Barbecue Sauce see page 137. Serve over Mock Mashed Potatoes
(page 218) and have a basket of Best Garlic Bread (page 26) ready.
Amount per serving, meatballs only (based on 4): 4.1 grams of carb,
31.8 grams of protein.

Barbecue Sauce

You do not need to be outdoors to enjoy this low-carb barbecue sauce
swirling around delicious meatballs. Makes about 3 cups.

PREPARATION TIME: 10 minutes. COOKING TIME: 1 hour.
SERVING SIZE: ½ cup. AMOUNT PER SERVING: 7.9 grams of carb, 3.1 grams
of protein. NUMBER OF SERVINGS: 5 to 6.

	CHO (g)	PRO (g)
1 cup canned, crushed tomatoes	12.0	4.0
2 cups stock or broth (page 80)	2.0	6.0
½ cup finely chopped onion	5.5	0.9
2 cloves garlic, minced (or ½ teaspoon garlic powder)	1.8	0
¼ cup white wine vinegar	0.5	0
2 teaspoons hickory smoke liquid	6.0	0
4 packets Splenda sugar substitute (or to taste)	4.0	0
1 tablespoon chili powder	1.5	0.9
1 teaspoon Dijon-style mustard	0.5	0.5
2 tablespoons Worcestershire sauce	6.0	0
salt to taste	0	0
freshly ground black pepper to taste	0	0
Total	*39.8*	*12.3*

Combine all the ingredients in a medium saucepan and simmer on
very low while you prepare the meatballs. When the meatballs are
browned, add sauce to skillet or casserole dish. Whether you cook
these in the skillet or oven, cook meatballs in sauce, stirring occasionally, over low heat (300°F) for 45 minutes to an hour.

Chili Con Carne with Black Soybeans

Read about Baked Black Soybeans on page 212 and find out about the great little black soybean that makes this and other bean dishes possible. One cup of regular high-carb chili has about 30.0 to 35.0 grams of carb. This chili—and it is quick and easy to fix—has 7.1 grams of carb in 1 cup (so go a little overboard if you are really hungry). Since this chili freezes well, you might want to cook the whole batch even if you need much less. Serve the chili with grated cheddar cheese and sour cream, if you like. Chips, plain or spicy (pages 197–98), go exceptionally well with it. You can cook the chili on the stovetop or put in a deep 4-quart casserole dish and bake it.

PREPARATION TIME: 20 to 25 minutes. COOKING TIME: 1½ hours.
SERVING SIZE: 1⅓ cup. AMOUNT PER SERVING: 7.1 grams of carb, 28.4 grams of protein. NUMBER OF SERVINGS: 8 to 9.

		CHO (g)	PRO (g)
2	cans (15 ounces each) black soybeans, drained and rinsed	22.4	48.4
3	tablespoons olive oil	0	0
3	tablespoons butter	0	0
½	cup chopped onion	5.5	0.9
2	pounds lean ground beef	0	160.0
3	tablespoons chili powder (or to taste)	4.5	0
	salt to taste (about 1 teaspoon)	0	0
	freshly ground black pepper	0	0
14½	ounces canned tomatoes, diced, with liquid	10.5	3.5
4	tablespoons tomato paste	10.0	4.0
3½	cups stock or broth (see page 80)	3.5	10.5
	Total	*56.4*	*227.3*

Have ready a large, heavy saucepan with lid or a Dutch oven. The alternate choice is to preheat the oven to 325°F and butter or oil a large, deep, ovenproof casserole dish. A cover is needed for this dish (aluminum foil is okay).

Put the soybeans in the bottom of the saucepan or casserole you intend to use for cooking.

Heat the skillet on medium heat and add about one-third of the olive oil and butter. When the butter foams (do not let it brown), add the onion and sauté until lightly browned. Add the sautéed onion to the black soybeans. Keep the skillet hot. Add the remaining fats. Cook the ground beef until lightly browned. Add the chili powder, salt, and pepper, and cook for another 2 or 3 minutes, stirring constantly. Add the tomatoes, tomato paste, and stock or broth. Stir until well mixed. Transfer the meat sauce to the saucepan or casserole dish. Stir to combine.

Simmer or bake the chili for about 1½ hours. If you cook it on the stovetop, stir now and then. If the chili is too thick for your liking, add a little water or stock. Adjust seasonings and serve. (This gets even better the next day.)

Variation: Slow-Cooked Chili Con Carne

The night before you want to slow cook, follow the directions for making Chili Con Carne on page 138, but add only 2 cups of stock or broth. Hold sauce in fridge overnight. Put sauce in the slow cooker in the morning. Set cooker to low and cook for 8 or 10 hours, or follow manufacturer's directions.

Caraway Beef Stew

What's better on a cold winter's day than a hot, bubbling pot of stew? This recipe is a spicy rendition on that old favorite. Pair it with a salad, if you like, and a warm loaf of Gourmet Rye Bread (page 36) for an easy supper, or serve it with Supreme Pasta (page 172). If you're in a maintenance phase of weight reduction and health recovery, you could even save room for Low-Carb Rhubarb Cobbler (page 287) or Creamy Berry Pie (page 285) for dessert. You can make the dish the day before; it gets even better reheated. It can be multiplied easily.

PREPARATION TIME: 20 minutes. BAKING TIME: 1½ to 2 hours.
SERVING SIZE: ⅙ total yield. AMOUNT PER SERVING: 11.8 grams of carb, 42.2 grams of protein. NUMBER OF SERVINGS: 6.

		CHO (g)	PRO (g)
3	tablespoons coconut oil	0	0
3	pounds beef chuck, cut into 1-inch cubes	0	240.0
2	tablespoons Hungarian sweet paprika	3.6	1.8
1	tablespoon caraway seeds	2.1	1.2
1	tablespoon dried marjoram	0.9	0
2	teaspoons salt	0	0
10	small yellow onions, sliced	52.5	8.2
½	cup dry red wine	2.0	0
1	tablespoon lemon juice (about ½ lemon)	1.3	0
1	tablespoon Wondra flour	5.8	0.8
1	tablespoon tomato paste	2.5	1.0
	parsley sprig	0	0
	Total	*70.7*	*253.0*

In a large stew pot or Dutch oven, heat the coconut oil. Add the meat all at once, turning until slightly browned on all sides.

In a small bowl, combine the paprika, caraway seeds, marjoram, and salt. Add one-half of this mixture to the stew pot and stir to blend.

Add the onions, red wine, and half of the lemon juice to the stew meat. Stir to blend. Simmer, uncovered, stirring occasionally, until the meat is tender, approximately 1½ to 2 hours.

Remove ½ cup liquid from the stew pot and put it in a small jar. Combine this liquid with the remaining spice mixture and lemon juice. Add the flour and tomato paste and stir until smooth. Return this mixture to the stew pot, stir to blend, and simmer about 15 minutes more. Ladle into bowls and garnish with a sprig of parsley for color.

Low-Carb French Dip Sandwich

If you like the classic French dip, now you can have it again and still be healthy—with low-carb Magic Rolls (page 22). It's a great way to utilize leftover beef roast or steaks. Plan ahead and save juice from a roast that is being cooked. Add a steamed vegetable or green salad and dinner will be ready in no time.

PREPARATION TIME: 15 minutes (with Magic Rolls on hand).
SERVING SIZE: ½ total yield. AMOUNT PER SERVING: 6.2 grams of carb, 37.3 grams of protein. NUMBER OF SERVINGS: 2.

	CHO (g)	PRO (g)
4 Magic Rolls, heated and crisp (page 22)	10.8	22.8
butter to add to broth (optional)	0	0
salt to taste	0	0
freshly ground black pepper	0	0
butter (for rolls) if desired	0	0
6 ounces very thinly sliced, lean, cooked roast beef	0	51.0
½ cup broth from roast (see page 80)	0.5	1.5
Total	*11.3*	*75.3*

Preheat oven to 350°F. Warm meat by wrapping it in aluminum foil or putting it in a covered baking dish in oven for several minutes. Heat broth in microwave or on stovetop. Fill small, individual bowls with hot broth for dipping. See page 80 for information about extending or making stock or broth, if the amount from the roast is insufficient. Put meat on hot rolls (buttered, if desired) and season with salt and pepper at serving time.

Low-Carb Beef Stroganoff

This is one of the many quick and easy beef recipes that tastes fabulous with minimal effort thanks largely to sour cream. You can fix this meal in less than 30 minutes. Because it is so easy to do—and tastes absolutely delicious—it is a great meal to serve at your dinner parties. The dish is absolutely best if you use beef tenderloin. There is little waste, and you are better off serving smaller portions than using a lesser-quality meat in larger amounts. This is great served over any pasta from Chapter 6. Round off the meal with a crisp, zesty salad and Magic Rolls (page 22) and enjoy.

PREPARATION TIME: 25 minutes. COOKING TIME: 9–10 minutes.
SERVING SIZE: 1⅓ cups. AMOUNT PER SERVING: 5.4 grams of carb, 24.8 grams of protein. NUMBER OF SERVINGS: 4

		CHO (g)	PRO (g)
1½	pounds beef tenderloin, trimmed well	0	85.3
	salt to taste	0	0
	freshly ground pepper to taste	0	0
12	ounces small button mushrooms	12.0	8.0
2	tablespoons coconut oil	0	0
1	ounce butter	0	0
¾	cup stock or broth (see page 80)	0.8	2.3
2	teaspoons Wondra flour	3.8	0
¾	cup sour cream	4.8	3.6
2	tablespoons freshly chopped parsley (or small sprigs)	0	0
	Total	*21.4*	*99.2*

Pound meat thin. Cut in strips about ¼ inch wide and 2 inches long. Put on a large plate and sprinkle lightly with salt and pepper. If you have time, refrigerate meat for an hour or longer.

Wipe mushrooms clean with a damp paper towel. Trim off hard ends of stems.

Heat a large, heavy skillet on medium-high. Add the oil. Quickly brown the meat in the hot oil on both sides, about 2 minutes total. Remove meat to a holding plate. Add the butter to the skillet. Reduce heat to medium-low. Add the mushrooms and cook until tender, about 5 minutes. Add the beef stock and stir to loosen particles on the bottom of the skillet. Add the flour and stir into the broth. Simmer for about 2 minutes on low. Add the meat and the sour cream and heat through. Adjust seasoning, sprinkle with parsley, and serve immediately.*

Variation: Low-Carb Chicken Stroganoff

It is a real treat to make this meal with bite-size pieces of chicken breast. Use 4 skinless chicken breast halves. Wash and pat the chicken dry. Cut in bite-size chunks, not as thin as you slice the beef. Add the chicken pieces to the hot oil; stir and brown them. The chicken pieces need to be cooked through; it takes about 6 to 8 minutes, depending on size and heat. Do not overcook. Sprinkle the chicken with a little salt and freshly ground pepper while cooking. When the chicken is done, remove to a holding plate and follow the recipe.

Note: If you are not prepared to serve the meal promptly after you have added the flour and stirred the stock, remove the pan from the heat until you are. (If this is going to take longer than 30 minutes, refrigerate everything until you are ready.) Reheat mushrooms and stock in skillet until bubbly. Proceed with recipe.

Breaded Pork Chops

Juicy, tender pork chops with a breaded coating—what a treat, and you can do it quickly, too. Buy boneless sirloin chops (or use tenderloin). Bread them, brown them lightly in a skillet, and bake them in the oven. It is as simple as that. Use Bread Crumbs I (page 25) or gluten-free Bread Crumbs II (page 26) from Chapter 2. If you want, you can make a pan gravy to smother the chops (page 111). Serve over your choice of low-carb pasta (Chapter 6) or make Best Garlic Bread (page 26) or focaccia with garlic topping (see Chapter 6). Magic Rolls (page 22) will always do the job, too. Add a steamed vegetable or lively salad.

PREPARATION TIME: 15 minutes. BAKING TIME: 40 to 45 minutes.
SERVING SIZE: 1 pork chop. AMOUNT PER SERVING: 2.6 grams of carb, 30.4 grams of protein. NUMBER OF SERVINGS: 4.

	CHO (g)	PRO (g)
¾ cup Bread Crumbs I (page 22)	8.4	17.1
½ teaspoon garlic powder	1.2	0
1 tablespoon Parmesan cheese	0.3	3.0
1 egg, beaten	0.6	6.0
4 pork sirloin/tenderloin chops, 1 inch thick	0	95.6
2 tablespoons coconut oil or butter	0	0
Total	*10.5*	*121.7*

Preheat oven to 325°F. Lightly grease a medium-size ovenproof casserole or baking dish with butter or coconut oil.

In a small, shallow bowl, mix the bread crumbs with the garlic powder and Parmesan cheese. Put the beaten egg into another small, shallow bowl (or on a plate). Remove all fat from the chops; clean and pat dry. Dip each chop first in the egg, then in the bread-crumb mixture. Coat well. Place on a platter.

Heat a medium or large skillet on medium-low. Heat coconut oil or butter and add the chops when the fat is hot. Turn down heat and briefly fry the chops until lightly browned on both sides, about 2 or 3 minutes. Transfer the chops to the casserole dish and bake for about 40 to 45 minutes or until done. (Check doneness with an instant-read meat thermometer.) Make the pan gravy (page 111) while the chops are baking. Serve immediately.

Veal Stew

The delicate flavors of veal and mushrooms play an interesting coun-terpoint to the sharper ones of onion, garlic, and cloves. You'll be proud to serve this entree to your most demanding guests, paired with a serving of vegetables and some crusty Magic Rolls (page 22).

PREPARATION TIME: 30 minutes. COOKING TIME: 1½ hours.
SERVING SIZE: ⅙ total yield. AMOUNT PER SERVING: 12.4 grams of carb, 44.9 grams of protein. NUMBER OF SERVINGS: 6.

		CHO (g)	PRO (g)
3	pounds veal shoulder, cut into 1-inch cubes	0	248.9
1	medium onion, stuck with 3 cloves	11.0	2.0
1	clove garlic, sliced into 3 or 4 pieces	0.9	0
¼	teaspoon dried thyme	0.6	0
1	teaspoon salt	0	0
24	fresh mushroom caps	4.0	2.0
2	teaspoons fresh lemon juice	0.9	0
9	very small onions	47.3	7.3
2	egg yolks, beaten	0.6	5.6
1	tablespoon flour	5.8	0.8
½	cup heavy cream	3.3	2.5
4	tablespoons butter, melted (½ stick)	0	0
	Total	*74.4*	*269.1*

Put veal, onion stuck with cloves, garlic, thyme, and salt into a large stew pot or Dutch oven; add enough water to cover.

Cook over low heat for about 1½ hours, or until veal is tender.

In a separate saucepan, cook the mushroom caps in boiling water with 2 teaspoons lemon juice for 5 minutes. Remove the caps with a slotted spoon and reserve liquid. Poach the small onions in this mush-room water until just tender, about 8 to 10 minutes. Discard the water.

Beat the egg yolks (which are already beaten), flour, and cream together in a small bowl.

Remove ¼ cup of meat broth from the stew pot and place it in a small saucepan. Add the melted butter and the egg yolk–cream mix-ture to it and whisk to blend thoroughly. Cook the sauce down, but do not let it boil. Heap veal on a hot platter, surrounding the meat with the onions and mushrooms. Pour the sauce over the dish and serve.

Rosemary Leg of Lamb

A delicious and delicate blend of herbs makes this lamb a treat, either served hot with a Roasted Asparagus Salad (page 88) and Yellow Crookneck Squash Casserole (page 230) or sliced cold for great sandwiches or entree salads for lunch the next day.

PREPARATION TIME: 25 minutes (needs 8 hours or overnight marinating). BAKING TIME: 1 hour and 40 minutes.

SERVING SIZE: ⅙ total yield. AMOUNT PER SERVING: 2.4 grams of carb, 47.2 grams of protein. NUMBER OF SERVINGS: 6.

	CHO (g)	PRO (g)
3 pounds boneless leg of lamb	0	279.6
5 large sprigs fresh rosemary	0	0
HERB PASTE		
½ cup fresh rosemary	2.4	0.5
1 tablespoon fresh thyme	0.2	0
7 cloves garlic	6.5	1.3
1 tablespoon Dijon-style mustard	1.5	1.5
1 teaspoon salt	0	0
¾ teaspoon black pepper	0.8	0
6 tablespoons olive oil	0	0
SAUCE		
¼ cup dry red wine	1.0	0
1 teaspoon balsamic vinegar	0.7	0
1 teaspoon Dijon-style mustard	0.5	0.5
½ teaspoon salt	0	0
½ teaspoon pepper	0.5	0
Total	*14.1*	*283.4*

Make the herb paste in the blender by processing the rosemary, thyme, garlic, mustard, salt, and pepper. With the blender running, slowly add the olive oil. Blend until the mixture is a sauce consistency. If needed, stop the blender, scrape down the sides, then continue blending. Set aside.

Spread the leg of lamb open (if rolled and tied, cut twine and open). Place the meat in a glass baking dish large enough to lay it flat. Spread half of the herb paste on the top side of the meat. Turn the meat over and spread the remaining paste on the other side. Cover tightly and refrigerate for 8 hours or overnight.

Preheat oven to 425°F when you are ready to roast the lamb. Lightly oil a shallow glass baking dish.

Without removing the paste, roll up the lamb jelly-roll style, starting from the long side; tie with cooking twine at both ends and in the middle to hold it securely.

Put the 5 rosemary sprigs in the bottom of the baking dish. Set the leg of lamb on top of the sprigs. Roast the lamb at 425°F for 10 minutes. Reduce heat to 350°F and continue to roast for another 1½ hours. Transfer the lamb to a heatproof serving platter, cover, and allow to rest before carving.

Make the sauce by removing the rosemary sprigs from the roasting pan. On the stovetop, over medium-low heat, stir the red wine into the pan juices, scraping all brown bits that may cling to the pan. Begin to briskly whisk the liquid, adding the balsamic vinegar and mustard. Taste the sauce and add the salt and pepper as needed. Put the sauce in a gravy boat or sauce pitcher to serve over the lamb at the table.

GUIDELINES FOR COOKING GAME MEATS

Our thanks go to New West Foods, Inc., for contributing the following guidelines for cooking game meats. Although given for buffalo and ostrich, the same rules generally apply to cuts of venison, elk, and wild boar, and their ground products, as well. See the "Mail-Order Sources" section for information on contacting New West Foods.

- All steaks should be rinsed under cool tap water and patted dry before seasoning, marinating, or cooking.
- Thaw all buffalo or ostrich meat in the refrigerator and not at room temperature.
- Meat can be cooked from the frozen, semifrozen, or thawed state.
- When cutting meat into strips, cut when meat is semifrozen if possible.
- Always marinate steaks covered in the refrigerator and not at room temperature.
- Buffalo or ostrich meat will get tough when overcooked. Steaks may benefit from basting with a light oil, marinade, or sauce prior to grilling to maintain moisture.
- Most meats can be reheated one time.
- *Broiling or grilling:* Broil meat 3–5 inches from heat.

    For 1-inch-thick cuts, broil 3 to 5 minutes per side for rare; 5 to 7 minutes per side for medium.

    For 1½-inch-thick cuts, broil 5 to 6 minutes per side for rare; 7 to 9 minutes per side for medium.

    For 2-inch-thick cuts, broil 7 to 10 minutes per side for rare; 10 to 13 minutes per side for medium.

- Cooking times may vary.
- Cook all ground meat to 165°F and maintain at 140°F. Ground meat is best prepared from a thawed state to ensure even and thorough cooking.

Grilled Bourbon Buffalo Steaks

Here's a dish for the cowboy and cowgirl in all of us. For the guy or gal who was born too late to rope and ride at the roundup, sleep on a bedroll under a canopy of stars, and grill a fresh buffalo steak over the open fire, this dish is the next best thing. It deserves to be eaten with a flavorful hearty vegetable such as Roasted Asparagus Salad (page 88) or Elegant Eggplant Parmigiana (page 222), a warm loaf of Gourmet Rye Bread (page 36), and a shot of good bourbon. But don't fear—a simple Caesar Salad, Best Garlic Bread (page 26), and a bottle of Zinfandel will work well for the city slickers. The recipe doubles easily for bigger crowds—all that limits you is the size skillet you have available for finishing the steaks.

PREPARATION TIME: 5 minutes. TOTAL COOKING TIME: 12 minutes.

SERVING SIZE: 1 steak. AMOUNT PER SERVING: 4.3 grams of carb, 36.9 grams of protein. NUMBER OF SERVINGS: 4.

	CHO (g)	PRO (g)
4 buffalo strip loin steaks (6 ounces each, 1 inch thick)	0	144.0
1 teaspoon garlic salt	0.5	0
2 tablespoons freshly ground black pepper	6.0	1.8
2 tablespoons butter	0	0
2 small yellow onions, diced	10.5	1.6
¼ cup Jack Daniel's or other good bourbon	0	0
Total	*17.0*	*147.4*

Light grill and let the grill or the coals get medium hot.

Rinse the steaks under cool tap water and pat them dry with paper towels. Dust both sides of each steak lightly with garlic salt and press the pepper into both sides of the meat. Place steaks on the grill. Grill for 2 to 3 minutes on each side and remove from heat.

To finish the steaks, melt butter and sauté onion in a skillet until tender and translucent, just starting to become golden. Add the steaks to the pan with the onions, then add the bourbon. Finish cooking steaks another total 3 to 5 minutes, turning once, for medium-rare to medium. Do not overcook.

Variation: Broiled Buffalo Steaks with Red Pepper Sauce

	CHO (g)	PRO (g)
2 buffalo ribeye steaks (8 ounces each)	0	80.0
½ teaspoon salt	0	0
1 teaspoon black pepper	1.0	0
SAUCE		
1 tablespoon butter	0	0
3 medium tomatoes, seeded and chopped	11.0	3.0
2 canned roasted red peppers, seeded and chopped	6.0	0
¾ teaspoon dried oregano	0.3	0
½ teaspoon garlic powder	1.2	0
½ teaspoon paprika	0.3	0
¼ teaspoon cayenne pepper	0	0
Total	*19.9*	*83.0*

Preheat oven broiler to high (500°F).

To make the sauce, melt the butter in a saucepan and add the tomatoes and peppers, cooking until the tomatoes are soft. Stir frequently. Add the oregano, garlic powder, paprika, and cayenne. Continue to cook and stir for 3 to 5 minutes, until the sauce thickens. Keep warm over very low heat while the steaks cook.

Rinse the steaks under cool water and pat them dry with paper towels. Sprinkle with salt and pepper. Lightly grease a broiling rack and pan with coconut oil. Place the steaks on the broiling rack about 3 to 5 inches from the heat. Broil for 6 to 8 minutes, turning halfway through the broiling time. For 1-inch steaks, about 6 minutes will yield a rare steak and 8 minutes will yield a medium-rare steak. Top the hot steaks with the red pepper sauce and serve.

Venison Sausage Stew

In cold weather, nothing is more comforting than a savory stew, piping hot and aromatic. You'll find this one so warm and filling that all you'll need to add is a green salad and some warm Rye Bread with Caraway (page 36), Best Garlic Bread (page 26), or Hearty Country Rolls (page 37) for a complete dining experience—oh, and a glass of a full-bodied red wine, if you like.

PREPARATION TIME: 20 minutes. COOKING TIME: 2½ hours.
SERVING SIZE: ¼ total yield. AMOUNT PER SERVING: 11.0 grams of carb, 16.6 grams of protein. NUMBER OF SERVINGS: 4.

		CHO (g)	PRO (g)
2	tablespoons coconut oil	0	0
1	medium onion, chopped	10.9	1.7
2	medium carrots, chopped	12.0	2.0
2	ribs celery, chopped	1.6	0.6
8	ounces whole white mushrooms, quartered	8.0	4.0
1	teaspoon salt	0	0
1	teaspoon freshly ground black pepper	1.0	0
1	teaspoon dried thyme	0.6	0
1	teaspoon garlic powder	2.3	0.5
1	bay leaf	0.3	0
1	teaspoon Worcestershire sauce	0.3	0
2	packages venison sausage (about 16 ounces)	3.6	55.3
½	cup heavy cream (optional)	3.2	2.4
	Total	*43.8*	*66.5*

In a Dutch oven or heavy soup pot, melt 1 tablespoon of the coconut oil. Add onion and sauté until translucent. Add the carrots, celery, and mushrooms and sauté for a couple of minutes, stirring to prevent sticking. Sprinkle the salt, pepper, thyme, and garlic powder over the cooking vegetables. Crumble in the bay leaf. Add 3 cups of water. Cover and cook over low heat for 2 hours.

Cut the sausages into bite-size pieces. Melt 1 tablespoon of coconut oil in a skillet; sauté the sausage pieces until well browned. Remove from heat and set aside. About 15 to 20 minutes before the vegetables are finished, add the venison sausage and Worcestershire sauce to the pot and continue to cook all together.

You can also add the cream now if you like a slightly thicker sauce.

Ostrich Patties in Mushroom Wine Sauce

Although an ostrich is a bird, its meat is quite red and extremely lean and flavorful. The sauce is so rich and savory, you'll want to serve it with a side dish of Mock Mashed Potatoes (page 218) or homemade Reduced-Carb Pasta (page 174) along with a colorful tossed garden salad. Like other red meats, ostrich pairs well with red wines, such as zinfandels, cabernets, or merlots. Once you try it, you'll be hooked, and although this recipe serves two, it will multiply easily so that you can treat your friends.

PREPARATION TIME: 10 minutes. COOKING TIME: 25 minutes.

SERVING SIZE: 1 patty. AMOUNT PER SERVING: 9.7 grams of carb, 49.5 grams of protein. NUMBER OF SERVINGS: 2.

	CHO (g)	PRO (g)
1 package ground ostrich meat (12 ounces)	0	91.5
½ cup half and half	5.2	3.6
2 tablespoons minced onion	2.0	0
4 tablespoons coconut oil	0	0
2 tablespoons butter	0	0
¾ cup dry red wine	3.0	0
½ cup heavy cream	3.2	2.4
1 tablespoon Worcestershire sauce	3.0	0
2 tablespoons dried parsley flakes	0	0
¾ cup fresh chopped mushrooms	3.0	1.5
Total	*19.4*	*99.0*

In a large bowl, mix together the ground ostrich meat, the half and half, and the onion. Shape into two large patties.

Heat the oil in a heavy skillet and brown the patties on both sides. Remove them and set aside to drain on several thicknesses of paper towels.

In the same skillet, melt the butter and add the wine, ¼ cup water, and heavy cream. Allow to thicken, stirring constantly. Add the Worcestershire sauce, parsley, and mushrooms and stir a moment or two. Return the patties to the skillet, cover, and simmer for 20 minutes, occasionally basting with the sauce. Serve immediately.

Breaded Halibut Baked in Sour Cream

This is one of the tastiest ways to fix halibut (or other white fish). No one will be sorry if it shows up on the menu often, especially during halibut season. For the cook, it is an easy, quick production. One condition must be met (as in all seafood) for this dish to be a huge success—the fish must be perfectly fresh or fresh frozen. Look for fish that is firm, white, and shiny.

PREPARATION TIME: 20 minutes (plus waiting time). BAKING TIME: 12 to 15 minutes.

SERVING SIZE: 1 halibut steak. AMOUNT PER SERVING: 5.2 grams of carb, 36.3 grams of protein. NUMBER OF SERVINGS: 4.

	CHO (g)	PRO (g)
8 ounces dry white wine	0	0
4 skinned and boned halibut steaks or fillets (5 ounces each)	0	118.0
1 teaspoon coarse or Kosher salt	0	0
1 cup Bread Crumbs I (page 25)	11.2	22.8
½ cup Basic Mayonnaise (page 239)	0	0
½ cup sour cream	4.0	3.2
½ cup finely chopped onion	5.5	0.9
2 teaspoons finely chopped fresh dill	0	0
4 sprigs of parsley or cilantro		
Total	*20.7*	*144.9*

Preheat oven to 350°F. Butter four individual fish-shaped casseroles (about 8 inches long). Sprinkle about a teaspoon of wine on top of the butter. Set aside.

Wash fish and pat dry with paper towels. Soak the fish in the remainder of the white wine mixed with the salt for about 30 minutes.

Put the bread crumbs in a shallow bowl. Dip the wet halibut steaks in the bread crumbs, coating them thoroughly. Transfer the steaks to the buttered, individual casserole dishes.

Mix the mayonnaise, sour cream, onion, and dill. Put one-quarter of this mixture over each of the halibut steaks. Bake the fish for about 12 to 15 minutes or until tender. Garnish with parsley or cilantro. Serve immediately.

Easy Salmon Casserole

You can make this dish with leftover baked salmon or with canned salmon. (The baked salmon will taste superb; the canned salmon will be very good.) This is airy, almost like a soufflé. Unlike a soufflé, this dish will not collapse when you serve it. It is quick to toss together, too.

PREPARATION TIME: 15 minutes. BAKING TIME: 35 to 45 minutes.
SERVING SIZE: ¼ total yield. AMOUNT PER SERVING: 3.8 grams of carb, 32.4 grams of protein. NUMBER OF SERVINGS: 4.

		CHO (g)	PRO (g)
16	ounces cooked or canned salmon	0	92.0
2	eggs	1.2	12.0
½	cup light cream	3.2	2.4
½	cup Bread Crumbs I (page 25)	5.4	11.4
2	tablespoons grated onion	2.0	0
1	tablespoon lemon juice	1.3	0
½	teaspoon Worcestershire sauce	0.5	0
¼	cup freshly minced parsley		
	(or 1 teaspoon dried)	0.4	0
	salt to taste (about ½ teaspoon or less)	0	0
	freshly ground black pepper to taste	0	0
3	tablespoons butter	0	0
¼	cup grated Parmesan cheese	1.0	11.9
	Total	*15.0*	*129.7*

Preheat oven to 375°F. Lightly oil or butter an ovenproof baking or casserole dish.

Flake the salmon (if you are using canned salmon, carefully drain it and discard all skin and bones) and put it in the casserole dish.

In a medium mixing bowl, beat the eggs until well combined and smooth. Add the cream. Mix well. Stir in the bread crumbs, onion, lemon juice, Worcestershire sauce, and parsley. Add salt and pepper. Add this mixture to the salmon and stir gently. Dot the casserole with butter and sprinkle the grated Parmesan cheese over it. Bake, uncovered, for about 35 to 45 minutes or until the top is nicely browned.

Salmon Cakes

Yummy treats for lunch, brunch, or supper, these make a nutritious meal you can throw together in a short time. Best with leftover salmon, but you can also use canned salmon. (If you make these salmon cakes really small, about an inch or so, you can use them as appetizers as well.) Serve with a green salad or with Cucumber Dill Sauce (page 246), Quickie Mushroom Sauce (page 249), or Quickie Lemon Sauce (page 250).

PREPARATION TIME: 15 minutes (plus waiting time). COOKING TIME: 8 minutes.

SERVING SIZE: 2 cakes. AMOUNT PER SERVING: 7.8 grams of carb, 36.9 grams of protein. NUMBER OF SERVINGS: 2.

	CHO (g)	PRO (g)
8 ounces cooked salmon (or 7¾ ounces canned salmon)	0	46.0
½ cup minced green (and white) onion	2.4	0.9
1 egg, beaten	0.6	6.0
½ cup Eden black soybeans, drained and rinsed	3.2	6.9
2 tablespoons light or heavy cream	0.8	0.6
salt to taste (about ½ teaspoon)	0.0	0.0
freshly ground black pepper	0	0
1 teaspoon freshly minced dill or ¼ teaspoon dried dill	0	0
½ cup Bread Crumbs I (page 25)	5.6	11.4
¼ cup unprocessed wheat bran	3.0	2.0
3 tablespoons coconut or olive oil	0	0
Total	*15.6*	*73.8*

Flake salmon (or drain canned salmon and flake). (Salmon should not have any skin or bones.) Put the salmon in a mixing bowl.

Combine the salmon, onion, egg, cream, salt, pepper, and dill. Add this mixture to the salmon along with the bread crumbs. Mix well. Refrigerate the mixture for about 20 to 30 minutes. Shape eight patties.

Heat a heavy skillet on medium to medium-low. Melt butter and heat until foamy (do not brown). Add the salmon cakes to the butter and cook until golden brown on both sides (about 4 minutes on each side). Reduce heat if the cakes brown too quickly.

Whitefish and Zucchini Bake

This cheesy one-dish fish and veggie meal needs only a crisp garden salad and a slice of warm Black Soybean Bread (page 29) and butter to make a great meal. The recipe can be multiplied easily for larger crowds and makes a great, easy buffet supper.

PREPARATION TIME: 15 minutes. BAKING TIME: 20 to 28 minutes.
SERVING SIZE: ¼ total yield. AMOUNT PER SERVING: 3.4 grams of carb, 34.8 grams of protein. NUMBER OF SERVINGS: 4.

		CHO (g)	PRO (g)
4	skinned whitefish fillets (about 5 ounces each)	0	108.2
1	teaspoon salt	0	0
1	teaspoon black pepper	1.0	0
1½	ounces butter	0	0
½	cup grated Parmesan cheese	2.0	23.8
3	small zucchini, sliced into thin rounds	10.0	6.9
¼	cup freshly chopped parsley	0.4	0.4
1	tablespoon olive oil	0	0
	Total	*13.4*	*139.3*

Preheat oven to 375°F. Generously butter a shallow baking dish.

Wash the fish and pat dry with paper towels. Arrange fillets in the buttered dish. Sprinkle evenly with salt and pepper and half of the grated cheese. Arrange the zucchini rounds over the fish in a single layer and salt and pepper lightly.

Mix the remaining cheese with the parsley and sprinkle this mixture over the zucchini layer. Dot with the butter.

Bake for 15 minutes. Remove from the oven and drizzle the olive oil evenly over the top. Return to the oven and cook another 5 to 8 minutes until golden brown.

Breaded Sole

Sole tends to become watery when cooked, but it has a delicious, delicate flavor and is economical, too. The breading gives it a little more body and improves the flavor. Make sure to buy perfectly fresh fish.

PREPARATION TIME: 15 minutes. COOKING TIME: 6 minutes (if the fish is cooked in two stages, double time).

SERVING SIZE: ¼ total yield. AMOUNT PER SERVING: 3.6 grams of carb, 35.5 grams of protein. NUMBER OF SERVINGS: 4.

		CHO (g)	PRO (g)
20	ounces fillets of sole (weight after discards)	0	107.0
1½	cup Bread Crumbs I (page 25)	11.2	22.8
2	eggs, beaten	1.2	12.0
4	tablespoons olive oil (or more)	0	0
1½	ounces butter (or more)	0	0
	sprigs of parsley or cilantro	0	0
4	lemon wedges	2.0	0
	Total	*14.4*	*141.8*

Preheat oven to 275°F. For this meal, it is a good idea to heat the serving plates and serve the sole on hot plates. There are many pieces of sole. They may crowd even two skillets if cooked simultaneously. Be prepared to cook fish in two stages. Keep warm in oven.

Clean fish by cutting the very thin ends off the fillets (cook them separately for your dog or cat). Wash the fish and dry with paper towels.

Put the bread crumbs on one large plate and the eggs in a large, shallow bowl. First, dip the sole in the egg, then coat thoroughly with bread crumbs. Place the coated pieces on a platter and set aside.

Heat two large, heavy skillets on medium-low. When the skillets are hot, add the olive oil and butter. When the butter bubbles (do not brown), put the sole in the skillet and cook for about 3 minutes on each side or until done—the fish should be flaky and opaque. Do not overcook. If you cannot cook all the pieces at once, keep the first batch warm in the oven. When you are about ready to serve, melt a little butter in the skillet and brown lightly. Drizzle over the cooked sole. Garnish with parsley or cilantro and lemon wedges.

Variation: Other Breaded Fish

You are by no means limited to sole. You can use any white fish, such as bass, grouper, monkfish, cod, orange roughy, red snapper, or whiting. Just follow the recipe. You may need to cook the fish up to 4 to 5 minutes on each side, depending on the size of the fish. You can vary the size of the pieces, depending on the fish of your choice.

Tuna Crunch

These easy, tasty, nutty fish burgers are sure to become a household favorite. You can eat them burger style on a Magic Roll (page 22) with lettuce, tomato, low-carb tartar sauce (page 239), and pickles, or simply paint a big leaf of lettuce with mayo, mustard, and dill pickle relish and wrap them up. Either way, they go well with a side of Avocado Slaw (page 89) and a big glass of iced tea.

PREPARATION TIME: 20 minutes. COOKING TIME: 6 to 8 minutes.

SERVING SIZE: 2 patties. AMOUNT PER SERVING: 2.1 grams of carb, 28.5 grams of protein. NUMBER OF SERVINGS: 2.

		CHO (g)	PRO (g)
1	can water-packed light tuna (6 ounces)	0	42.1
2	green (and white) onions, minced	1.0	0
2	tablespoons freshly chopped parsley	0	0
½	teaspoon salt	0	0
¼	teaspoon dried thyme	0.2	0
⅛	teaspoon freshly ground black pepper	0.1	0
12	pecan halves, broken into small pieces	1.7	2.8
2	eggs, slightly beaten	1.2	12.0
2	tablespoons coconut oil	0	0
	Total	*4.2*	*56.9*

Open and drain the can of tuna. In a small mixing bowl, flake the fish. Add the onion, parsley, salt, thyme, pepper, and pecan pieces; stir well to combine. Add the eggs and blend thoroughly.

Heat the coconut oil in a heavy skillet. Drop the tuna mixture by heaping tablespoons (about one-quarter of the mixture) into the skillet. Flatten slightly with a spatula or back of a spoon. You should have four patties of about equal size. Sauté about 3 or 4 minutes and turn, cooking until browned on both sides. Drain on absorbent paper towels and serve immediately.

Tuna Casserole

A can or two of solid white tuna, mixed with a few ingredients and thrown into a casserole dish, comes out tasting like a well-planned meal. Add a fresh green salad and Magic Rolls (page 22) and dinner is served.

PREPARATION TIME: 20 minutes. BAKING TIME: 35 to 45 minutes.
SERVING SIZE: ¼ total yield. AMOUNT PER SERVING: 6.1 grams of carb, 29.6 grams of protein. NUMBER OF SERVINGS: about 4.

		CHO (g)	PRO (g)
2	6-ounce cans albacore tuna in olive oil or water, drained (10 ounces of tuna meat)	0	74.0
2	tablespoons olive oil or coconut oil	0	0
½	cup chopped onion	5.5	0.9
10	large, black, canned olives, chopped fine, or 5–6 fresh cured olives, such as Kalamata	3.0	0
1½	cups finely chopped celery	3.6	1.5
1	tablespoon drained and crushed capers	1.0	0
½	teaspoon garlic powder	1.2	0
2	teaspoons dried basil	1.4	0
	salt to taste	0	0
	freshly ground black pepper to taste	0	0
½	cup Bread Crumbs I (page 25)	5.6	11.4
3	egg yolks, beaten	0.6	5.6
⅔	cup heavy cream	4.2	3.2
⅓	cup stock or broth (page 80)	0.3	1.0
½	cup grated Parmesan cheese (or cheese of choice)	2.0	23.8
2	tablespoons butter (¼ of one stick)		
	Total	*28.4*	*119.4*

Preheat oven to 325°F. Lightly butter or oil a medium baking pan or ovenproof casserole dish.

Put tuna in a large mixing bowl; break up into smaller pieces.

Preheat a heavy skillet on medium. Add the oil to the hot skillet. Briefly sauté the onion, just until translucent. Add the olives, celery, capers, garlic powder, and basil, and cook for about 2 minutes. Season with the salt and pepper. Add the bread crumbs. Stir this mixture lightly into the tuna.

In a medium-size mixing bowl, beat the cream into the egg yolks (which are already beaten). Add the broth and beat again until mixed. Pour over the casserole. Sprinkle with the Parmesan cheese. Dot with the butter. Bake the casserole, uncovered, for 35 to 45 minutes or until the top is lightly browned.

Baked Tuna Burgers

These are a huge success yet require minimal effort to fix. You need Magic Rolls, hamburger bun size, on page 22 in Chapter 2. (This is one of many good reasons to bake ahead and keep a supply of the rolls on hand in the freezer.) Serve for lunch, brunch, or even as a light dinner.

PREPARATION TIME: 15 minutes. BAKING TIME: 15 to 20 minutes.
SERVING SIZE: 2 burgers. AMOUNT PER SERVING: 9.2 grams of carb, 39.3 grams of protein. NUMBER OF SERVINGS: 2.

	CHO (g)	PRO (g)
4 Magic Rolls, hamburger bun size (page 22)	16.4	34.0
6 ounce can albacore tuna in olive oil or water, drained	0	37.0
4 tablespoons finely chopped chives*	0.4	0
4 tablespoons finely minced celery	0.6	0
2 tablespoons Basic Mayonnaise (page 239)	0	
¼ cup grated cheddar cheese	0.4	7.1
1 tablespoon sour cream	0.5	0.4
salt to taste (about ¼ teaspoon)	0	0
freshly ground black pepper to taste	0	0
4 teaspoons butter	0	0
Total	*18.3*	*78.5*

Preheat oven to 325°F or 350°F. Tear off four 12- by 12-inch pieces of aluminum foil.

Slice the tops of the Magic Rolls and scoop out as much of the interior as you can. Set each roll on a square of aluminum foil.

Put the tuna in a small or medium mixing bowl and flake. Add the chives and celery to the tuna. Combine the mayonnaise, cheese, and sour cream. Add to the tuna. Add the salt and pepper and mix together.

Put equal amounts of filling in each roll. Dot each filling with a pat of butter. Replace roll tops (push firmly in place). Wrap each roll in foil, gathering the four corners loosely on top (air needs to be able to escape). Set the rolls on a cookie sheet or in a cake pan. Bake for about 15 to 20 minutes. Serve immediately.

---

* Fresh chives are better than dried. If you don't have chives, use finely minced green onions. (If you do not want to use any onions, the burgers will still taste very good.)

Variation: Baked Tuna Waffle   *(gluten-free)*

A baked tuna waffle is another great treat you do not see every day.
And it is gluten-free. Follow the recipe for Baked Tuna Burgers on
page 161. Prepare the filling as directed. Use one serving of Basic
Waffles (page 53) instead of the rolls (four 4-inch square waffles or
two 7- or 8-inch round waffles). For bigger appetites you might want
to make an extra serving to be split between two people. Place the filling between two waffles (or waffle halves). Use aluminum foil for
wrapping. Dot the top of the waffle burger with the butter. Carb and
protein counts remain essentially the same.

Scampi

This dish is, well, divine. Once you cook and serve this meal, you and everyone else will be hooked. Buy shrimp frozen—this is how most shrimp are delivered to stores, anyway. Avoid buying shrimp that has already been thawed for the store display. Put them in cold water to thaw when you are close to cooking them. Do the peeling (and deveining, if the shrimp are not already deveined) before the shrimp are fully thawed. Keep the tails attached. Buy medium or large shrimp (20 to 32 or so to the pound)—they are easier to peel. All you need to go with this dish is a small green salad and crisp Magic Rolls (page 22). For just a little more work, you can make a batch of Best Garlic Bread (page 26) and have a dinner that is out of this world.

PREPARATION TIME: 15 to 20 minutes. COOKING TIME: 15 minutes.
SERVING SIZE: ½ total yield. AMOUNT PER SERVING: 5.9 grams of carb, 34.5 grams of protein. NUMBER OF SERVINGS: 2.

	CHO (g)	PRO (g)
⅓ cup olive oil	0	0
⅓ cup fresh lemon juice	7.0	0
⅓ cup dry white wine	0.6	0
1 pound medium to large shrimp, shelled and deveined	3.0	69.0
6 tablespoons butter (¾ stick)	0	0
½ teaspoon garlic powder	1.2	0
salt to taste	0	0
freshly ground black pepper to taste	0	0
Total	*11.8*	*69.0*

Preheat oven to 250°F about 15 minutes before you plan to cook the shrimp. Put two individual ovenproof casserole dishes in the oven to have them piping hot at serving time. (You can use 8-inch-long oval casserole dishes for serving seafood if you desire.)

Put a large, heavy skillet on a cold burner. Add the olive oil, lemon juice, wine, and butter to the cold skillet. Heat very slowly on medium-low. When the sauce heats up, keep it at a very low simmer for about 5 minutes to fully blend the ingredients. Have the shrimp nearby. When you are ready to cook the shrimp, turn up the heat to medium-high. Add the garlic powder, salt, and pepper to the sauce and stir well; allow to sizzle for about 60 seconds. Add the shrimp and cook them, stirring constantly, for about 4 minutes or until pink. Put the shrimp in the heated casserole dishes and pour the sauce over them. Serve at once.

Tomato-Shrimp-Cheese Casserole

You'll love the Mediterranean flavors in this easy, quick casserole. It's practically a meal by itself; all you'll need is a garden salad and some Best Garlic Bread (page 26) to round out the plate. Even though it's seafood, the spicy tomato flavors pair well with light-bodied red wines, such as chianti or rioja.

PREPARATION TIME: 20 minutes. COOKING AND BAKING TIME: 25 to 30 minutes.

SERVING SIZE: ⅙ total yield. AMOUNT PER SERVING: 7.3 grams of carb, 27.1 grams of protein. NUMBER OF SERVINGS: 6.

		CHO (g)	PRO (g)
⅓	cup extra-virgin olive oil	0	0
1½	pounds large shrimp, shelled and deveined	6.2	138.2
1	medium yellow onion, coarsely chopped	7.5	1.3
3	cloves garlic, finely chopped or pressed	2.8	0.6
4	medium tomatoes, diced	17.4	4.2
1	teaspoon salt	0	0
½	teaspoon white pepper	0.5	0
¼	teaspoon dried thyme	0.2	0
5	tablespoons sherry vinegar	5.0	0
4	ounces feta cheese, crumbled	4.0	18.0
	Total	*43.6*	*162.3*

Preheat oven to 350°F. Oil an ovenproof casserole dish.

Preheat a large, heavy skillet on medium-high. Add the olive oil, but reserve 1 tablespoon for later use. Sauté the shrimp in the hot oil until almost done (just opaque). Take skillet off burner.

Preheat a smaller skillet. Add the reserved olive oil. Sauté the onion over medium heat until translucent; add the garlic and sauté for another minute. Add the tomatoes and simmer over low to medium heat for about 15 minutes more.

Add the tomato mixture to the shrimp and combine. Gently mix in the salt, pepper, thyme, and vinegar. Pour the shrimp and tomatoes into the casserole dish. Top with the feta cheese.

Bake for about 5 minutes or until cheese melts and the dish is warmed through. Serve immediately.

Variation: Tomato-Cheese-Scallop Casserole

This is a wonderful treat. Even though scallops have a mild flavor, they will hold their own baked in this quick and easy casserole. Buy about 24 ounces of sea scallops. Buy them fresh or solidly frozen, not from a display tray where the scallops may be thawed. Defrost them in the fridge or under cold running water. Drain and pat the scallops as dry as possible with paper towels. If you like, cut out the small whitish muscle that attaches the scallop to its shell. It is tougher than the rest but not by much. If the scallops are considerably larger than 1 inch, cut them in half. Follow the Tomato-Shrimp-Cheese Casserole on page 164, but use scallops instead of shrimp. Sauté the scallops on both sides, about 4 to 5 minutes total.

Breaded Scallops

Here is a new delight for folks on a low-carb diet: breaded sea scallops. Buy fresh scallops if possible. If you buy frozen scallops, buy them frozen or partially frozen rather than thawed in supermarket trays. Scallops cook quickly and can easily be served to guests.

PREPARATION TIME: 20 minutes. COOKING TIME: 4 to 8 minutes.

SERVING SIZE: 6 ounces scallops. AMOUNT PER SERVING: 7.3 grams of carb, 37.5 grams of protein. NUMBER OF SERVINGS: 4.

		CHO (g)	PRO (g)
24	ounces sea scallops	16.8	115.2
6	ounces dry white wine (optional)	0	0
1¼	cups Bread Crumbs I (page 25)	11.2	22.8
2	eggs, lightly beaten	1.2	12.0
4	tablespoons olive oil	0	0
4	tablespoons butter (½ stick)	0	0
4	tablespoons butter (optional)	0	0
	sprigs of parsley	0	0
4	lemon wedges (garnish)	0	0
	Total	*29.2*	*150.0*

Wash scallops and pat dry with paper towels. If you like, remove the small whitish muscle—it takes only a moment—that attaches the scallop to its shell. It is just slightly tougher than the rest of the meat but certainly acceptable. Put the scallops in an optional marinade of wine (mix with water if needed to cover scallops) for 30 minutes to 1 hour.

Preheat the oven to 250°F to keep dinner plates warm. (This is optional but adds a nice touch to the meal.)

Put the bread crumbs in one shallow bowl and the eggs in another. Dip scallops in the egg first, then coat thoroughly with the bread crumbs. Place the coated scallops on a platter and set aside.

Heat a large, heavy skillet on medium-low, more on the low side. Add the olive oil and butter. When the butter bubbles (do not brown), put the scallops in the skillet and cook them for 2 to 3 minutes on each side or until done. The low-carb bread crumbs tend to darken more quickly than ordinary bread crumbs. Keep the heat a little on the low side (lower than you would normally) and watch closely that the coating stays light and golden (reduce heat further, if needed).

Keep heat under the skillet and move the scallops to the pre-warmed serving plates. Quickly add the optional butter to the hot skillet and stir until it turns slightly brown. Drizzle over the scallops. Garnish with the parsley and lemon wedges. Serve immediately.

6

PASTA, PIZZA, TORTILLAS, AND MORE—DELICIOUS LOW-CARB ITALIAN AND MEXICAN RECIPES

Ah . . . pasta: the ultimate in comfort food. Most veterans of traditional low-carb eating will confess to missing the experience of biting into a forkful of al dente fettuccine, enrobed in a creamy Alfredo sauce. And who doesn't fondly recall the steaming plates of ravioli, lasagna, and cheese-stuffed cannelloni in a pool of rich marinara sauce that we once enjoyed before health or weight concerns ruled out such high-carb pleasures?

If you've wistfully longed for your favorite pasta recipes, the wait is over. Boil the water, break out the pasta bowls, dust off the red-checkered tablecloth, and put on the Tony Bennett CD. Pasta—in almost all its forms—is back on the menu. Now, with one-third the carbs of the regular stuff, it's totally in sync with your low-carb lifestyle. Dress it up with creamy sauces, rich tomato sauces, meatballs, seafood, or chicken. Add a warm loaf of the delicious focaccia bread you'll find in this chapter, some good olive oil for dipping, a green salad, and a bottle of nice chianti, and enjoy the smells and tastes of the old country again.

And if you've missed your Friday night pizza and beer, no need to cry in your suds. In this chapter, you'll find easy-to-prepare recipes for savory pizza, hot from the oven, made with raised dough crusts, or a quick personal pan pizza version made on low-carb waffles (page 53). So pour yourself a light beer, toss a salad, and it's pizza night once again.

But if, like many veteran low-carbers, it's the *olé!* you've missed most, your luck has finally changed. In traditional low-carb cookbooks, making Mexican dishes to suit the low-carb lifestyle bordered on the impossible; modifying Mexican was hands-down the greatest challenge of all world cuisines. What's a taco, after all, with no shell? A burrito without a wrapper? An enchilada with no tortilla? Salsa, *queso,* or guacamole without the chips? Except for the occasional dietary vacation since you began your low-carb lifestyle, you've probably missed the cheesy, savory comfort of enchiladas, eschewed the warm, soft bean burritos, eaten the fajitas without the tortillas, and dipped your *queso* with pork rinds or jicama slices. But no more!

In this chapter, you'll find a full menu worthy of a Mexican cantina, beginning with low-carb corn and flour tortillas for making tacos, enchiladas, burritos, fajitas, nachos, and more, complete with a side of low-carb "rice" and refried beans! You'll learn how easy it is to make your own plain and spicy chips, as well as some of the best South-of-the-Border dips you've ever dipped your chip into: the World's Best Guacamole (page 199), Salsa Verde good enough to make you weep (page 202), spicy Chile Con Queso (page 200), and back on the table at long last . . . bean dip! And all so low in carb, you won't have to worry about saying *más por favor!*

LOW-CARB PASTA

You can eat pasta again! Real pasta. But who wants to make pasta? Oh the mess—crank out dough—or roll it out—dry it—and wait. Luckily, making this pasta is incredibly quick and easy—just 30 minutes from start to finish—if you use an electric mixer with a pasta-making attachment. It is possible that electric pasta machines may do the job; however, they cost as much as an electric mixer and are much less versatile. Any simple, manual pasta machine that uses templates also will do the job well. Avoid machines that require the dough to be run between rollers. You can make the pasta by hand, too, but the process takes about 30 minutes longer. Although you can lay out the pasta to dry, it works well to cook the pasta the moment it is formed so that it goes from the pasta maker (or after you have rolled it out) straight into simmering water. A few minutes later, you can serve it. The cooked pasta freezes well and can be thawed in the microwave for instant use. Pasta you buy in the store usually has from 31.0 to 37.0 grams of carb in 1 cup of cooked pasta; the recipes here have either 12.7 grams—the "high-carb" version—or 8.8 grams of carb in 1 cup. As easy as it is to make, there is no reason you cannot have pasta fairly often.

Supreme Pasta

PREPARATION TIME: 30 minutes. COOKING TIME: 2 or 3 minutes.
SERVING SIZE: ½ cup. AMOUNT PER SERVING: 6.2 grams of carb, 9.4 grams of
protein. NUMBER OF SERVINGS: 9.

	CHO (g)	PRO (g)
1 tablespoon olive oil	0	0
1 teaspoon salt	0	0
⅓ cup vital wheat gluten flour	7.7	34.8
½ cup soy protein powder	0	32.0
½ cup unbleached, all-purpose wheat (white) flour (or whole wheat, if you prefer)	46.5	6.0
4 egg yolks	1.2	11.2
5 tablespoons cold water	0	0
3 tablespoons butter (or as desired)	0	0
Total	*55.4*	*84.0*

Heat about 4 quarts of water in a large (6 quart or larger capacity) stockpot and bring to a lively simmer. (A large pot makes it easier to stir the pasta and keep water from boiling over.) Add the olive oil and salt to the water.

Attach the pasta maker to your electric mixer. (Follow pasta maker instructions.) If possible, locate the mixer within easy reach of the pot of simmering water on the stove because the pasta is transferred directly to the water.

Combine the wheat gluten flour, soy protein powder, and wheat (white) flour in a small mixing bowl. Stir well. Put the egg yolks and water in another small bowl and beat until smooth. Pour the eggs and water over the flour mixture and stir briefly with a fork. Take over by hand and knead the dough until it is firm, almost hard, and rather dry (it takes just moments). This kind of dough makes cleanup a breeze because it moves more easily through the pasta maker. If the dough is soft, it tends to cling to the insides of the pasta maker. Because egg yolks vary in volume, you may sometimes need to add a small amount of water to gather up all loose crumbs. If this happens, add cold water by the teaspoon to make sure the dough stays dry. If the dough gets too soft, add a bit of soy protein powder. When the dough is ready, twist off chunks of dough the size of small plums and stretch them into sausage-shaped pieces. Put these in a bowl and have them ready to go.

Start the pasta maker and drop a piece of dough in the hopper. It will be propelled along by the machine. As it disappears, add the next.

If a piece of dough fails to advance by itself, use the plunger that comes with the pasta maker. Keep adding new chunks of dough. This process takes just 2 or 3 minutes. The first pasta tends to be a little slow to extrude and may curl in the beginning but will straighten out soon. Tear or cut off pasta when it is the length you like, although you might find shorter lengths, about 4 inches, most practical.

Drop the bundle of pasta into the simmering water and stir it for a few seconds to separate the individual strands. As you do this, the next bundle of pasta may be ready to be cut off (also make sure you keep feeding the hopper). Repeat this cycle until the last pasta has emerged. As you add fresh pasta to the pot, the volume of the pasta keeps increasing, of course. When the last bundle is in the water, continue simmering the pasta for another 2 or 3 minutes and stir frequently as you do. The first pasta you drop in the water will simmer longer than subsequent bundles. This does not affect the quality of the pasta. You will, however, be stirring a fairly large batch of pasta—about 4 cups—by the time you come to the end, so it is a good idea to use a long-handled wooden spoon, 14 inches or so, to make stirring easy and safe.

Drain the pasta in a colander. Do not rinse. Let the water drip off as much as possible. Put the hot pasta in a large mixing bowl. Stir in the butter. The total yield of cooked pasta from this recipe is a little over 4 cups. The pasta is ready to be served immediately or you can keep it in the fridge for four to five days or freeze it. Thaw frozen pasta in a microwave or fridge; heat in microwave.

To make pasta by hand, you need to make a few changes. You need to soften the dough to make it more pliable so that it will be easy to roll out. When you combine the cold water and egg yolks, increase the water from 5 to 7 tablespoons. You can always add an extra teaspoon or so of water, but the dough should not be sticky. Sprinkle a little soy protein powder on a large cutting board (with kitchen towel beneath it). Divide the dough in six or seven chunks. Roll each into a large, thin sheet. Use protein powder as needed, but you won't need much; the dough will be easy to handle. Cut each sheet in pasta shapes (a pastry cutter works well for this). Stack the sheets after they have been cut. Drop the sheets, one by one, into the simmering water and stir for a few seconds after each addition to allow the pasta to separate. After adding the last sheet, simmer the pasta for another 2 minutes. Continue as directed for the pasta made in the pasta maker. The yield of pasta is an additional ½ cup.

---

* When you run the dough through the pasta maker, a small amount lodges behind the blade and stays there (about ⅔ ounce). You lose 2 grams of carb this way.

Variation: Reduced-Carb Pasta

Follow the directions for making Supreme Pasta on page 172, but increase the vital wheat gluten flour to ⅔ cup. Increase the soy protein powder to ⅔ cup. Reduce the wheat (white) flour to ¼ cup. Increase the cold water to 7 tablespoons for the dough going through the pasta maker and increase to 9 tablespoons for the handmade pasta. The yield of the reduced-carb pasta is almost 5 cups. Total carbs for the batch are 37.6 grams. Total protein is 112.3 grams. A ½ cup serving of pasta has 3.8 grams of carb and 11.2 grams of protein. Pasta made by hand yields 5½ cups.

Fettuccine Alfredo

This is one of the quickest meals to put together. An elegant meal (great for company) can be assembled in less than 45 minutes if you have prepared pasta on hand. If you have to make the pasta, add 30 minutes, or 60 minutes if you must make it by hand. Since pasta is the main component of this meal, you might want to increase an individual serving from the normal $\frac{1}{2}$ cup to $\frac{3}{4}$ cup. Serve with a fresh green salad. Best Garlic Bread (page 26) goes superbly with this.

PREPARATION TIME: 30 minutes. COOKING TIME: 2 minutes.
SERVING SIZE: $\frac{1}{4}$ total yield. AMOUNT PER SERVING: 10.9 grams of carb, 29.4 grams of protein. NUMBER OF SERVINGS: 4.

		CHO (g)	PRO (g)
3	cups Supreme Pasta (page 172)	36.6	56.4
8	tablespoons butter (1 stick)	0	0
1	cup grated Parmesan cheese*	5.0	59.5
$\frac{1}{3}$	cup heavy cream	2.1	1.6
2	tablespoons freshly chopped parsley	0	0
	Total	*43.7*	*117.5*

Prepare one recipe of Supreme Pasta or thaw frozen pasta if you have it on hand.

Cut the butter into eight pieces. Heat the pasta in the top of a double boiler over hot or simmering but not boiling water. When the pasta is heated through, add the butter, Parmesan cheese, and cream. Stir until melded into a uniform, velvety texture. Transfer to a heated serving bowl or individual plates. Sprinkle with parsley and serve.

---

* Quality of the cheese makes a big difference here. If possible, use an imported cheese and grate it yourself.

Note: If you decide to make the Fettuccine Alfredo with the Low-Carb Pasta (page 171), the carb count per serving will be 8.1 grams.

Pasta "Fried Rice"

If you miss fried rice, this substitute is a treat. With pasta being so easy to make, you can serve Pasta "Fried Rice" often to those who miss it, although almost anyone will like this meal. If you have pasta ready to go, it's a cinch to put together. This is a good recipe in which to use the Reduced-Carb Pasta (page 174). This pasta is almost as good as the Supreme Pasta (page 172). By the time you mingle pasta, eggs, onions, and other flavors, you probably won't know the difference. And with the reduced carb count, fried rice lovers can eat an extra-large portion. Served with a hearty salad, it's a meal in itself.

PREPARATION TIME: 25 minutes or less (add 30 minutes or 1 hour if you have to make the pasta). COOKING TIME: 15 minutes.

SERVING SIZE: 1½ cups. AMOUNT PER SERVING: 9.2 grams of carb, 23.3 grams of protein. NUMBER OF SERVINGS: 5.

		CHO (g)	PRO (g)
4	cups Reduced-Carb Pasta (page 174)	30.4	86.9
2	tablespoons olive oil or coconut oil	0	0
4	eggs, lightly beaten	2.4	24.0
½	cup chopped onion	5.5	0.9
1½	cups chopped scallions (green and white parts)	7.2	1.9
3	cloves garlic, minced (or 1 teaspoon garlic powder)	2.7	0.6
1	cup snow peas	4.0	2.0
2	tablespoons butter (or as desired)	0	0
	salt to taste	0	0
	freshly ground black pepper to taste	0	0
2	tablespoons soy sauce (or as desired)	3.0	0
	Total	*55.2*	*116.3*

On a large cutting board, cut the pasta into small pieces, approximately ½ to 1 inch long. If you want, use a mezzaluna to cut the pasta.

Heat a large, heavy skillet on medium-low heat. Add the oil. Pour the eggs in the hot oil and allow them to spread as you would for an omelet. Do not stir. As soon as the eggs are cooked on one side and show dryness on top (it takes about 1 minute), turn the whole sheet of eggs with a spatula and cook for about 30 seconds on the other side. Spread a double layer of paper towels on a large cutting board and put the eggs on it. Soak up excess fat and allow to cool for handling. To cut, remove the paper towels and roll the sheet of eggs as if you were making a jelly roll. Cut the roll into thin strips (⅓ inch or so). Next cut them the other way. You want pieces that are approximately 1 by ⅓ inch long, although it's okay if you want to make them a different size.

Add more oil to the skillet, if needed. Sauté the onion until it is almost translucent. Add the green onion and garlic and cook for about 1 minute. Add the snow peas and cook for about 3 minutes; keep snow peas crunchy. Reduce heat if necessary. Add the chopped pasta and heat through, stirring all the time. Add the butter. Add the eggs last and stir again until the meal is hot. Season with salt and pepper. Thin the soy sauce with a few drops of water and pour over the pasta. Stir. Serve and offer soy sauce at the table.

Variation: Pasta "Fried Rice" with Chicken

Follow the recipe for Pasta "Fried Rice" on page 176, but reduce the amount of pasta to 3½ cups. Add 1 cup of bite-size pieces of cooked chicken to the pan after the eggs have been cooked. Stir briefly and brown lightly; it takes about 1 minute. Remove the chicken from the pan and set aside. Continue with the recipe as directed. Then add the browned chicken together with the chopped egg and heat through. You can substitute cooked pork for the chicken. The directions are the same; the carb and protein counts are also virtually the same. A serving (based on five) has 9.0 grams of carb and 34.0 grams of protein.

Variation: Pasta "Fried Rice" with Shrimp

Buy ½ pound cooked salad or popcorn shrimp. If they are not freshly cooked but cooked and previously frozen, do not buy them thawed. If possible, smell the shrimp; they should not smell. Rinse the shrimp under cold water to thaw. Pat thoroughly dry with paper towels. Marinate the shrimp for a couple of hours in this mixture: 2 tablespoons soy sauce, 1 teaspoon ground ginger, ¼ cup white wine, 1 tablespoon olive oil, 1 packet Splenda sugar substitute. When you are ready to use the shrimp, drain and dry them; discard the marinade. Follow the recipe for Pasta "Fried Rice" with Chicken (above). Add the shrimp to the skillet instead of the chicken. A serving (based on five) has 10.5 grams of carb and 35.0 grams of protein.

Note: You can cook the Pasta "Fried Rice" in a wok, if you like. Follow the directions for cooking the meal in a skillet, but heat the wok to medium-high; brush lightly with 1 tablespoon of coconut oil (bottom and sides). Divide the beaten eggs in four portions and fry each separately. Stack the eggs and cut into strips when cool. Add a little more oil to the wok and quickly sauté the onion (about 1 minute); add the green onion and garlic and cook for a few seconds. Add the snow peas and cook for 1 minute. Add the pasta and eggs and heat through. Wok cooking uses much less oil. It is fast and requires close attention.

Low-Carb Lasagna

This will be a thrill for lovers of lasagna. It is not a quick meal to put together unless you have a meat sauce ready. But with a supply of Italian Meat Sauce (page 134) on hand in the freezer and perhaps a supply of some pasta, you can build the lasagna in a hurry. If you want to make a batch of lasagna-type noodles, prepare the pasta by hand and roll out the wide strips with a pastry wheel. With a pasta attachment, the most you will get is something resembling egg noodles. (Actually, once you cover the noodles with cheese and sauce, how wide they are may not be all that critical.)

PREPARATION TIME: 20 minutes (if you have pasta and sauce on hand).
  BAKING TIME: 25 to 35 minutes.
SERVING SIZE: ⅛ total yield. AMOUNT PER SERVING: 11.6 grams of carb, 34.0 grams of protein. NUMBER OF SERVINGS: 8

		CHO (g)	PRO (g)
4	cups Supreme Pasta (page 172)*	54.7	84.2
4	cups Italian Meat Sauce (page 134)	20.8	63.6
8	ounces thinly sliced whole-milk mozzarella cheese	5.6	49.6
1	cup grated Parmesan cheese	4.0	47.6
1	cup whole-milk ricotta cheese	7.6	27.6
½	cup grated Parmesan cheese	2.0	23.8
	Total	*94.7*	*296.4*

Preheat oven to 350°F just before you are ready to build the lasagna. Butter or oil a 13- by 9- by 2½-inch baking pan or ovenproof casserole dish.

Prepare or thaw Supreme Pasta (page 172), any shape. Put the pasta in a bowl.

Build the lasagna by spreading a third of the pasta evenly over the bottom of the baking pan. Pour 1⅓ cups of sauce over the pasta. Cover the sauce with a third of each of the three cheeses. Follow with a second layer of pasta and repeat the sequence: 1⅓ cups sauce and a third of each of the cheeses. Place the last bunch of pasta on top and top it with the remaining sauce and cheeses, in that order. Sprinkle with the ½ cup Parmesan cheese. (You can prepare this dish several hours earlier or even a day ahead; keep refrigerated.) Bake the lasagna for 25 to 35 minutes or until bubbly and lightly browned on top. Let the lasagna sit for about 15 to 20 minutes, covered to keep it warm, before cutting.

* You can use Reduced-Carb Pasta on page 174 instead of Supreme Pasta. It will save a total of 15.8 grams of carb and add 28.1 grams of protein. A single serving (based on eight) has 9.2 grams of carb and 36.6 grams of protein.

Deluxe Low-Carb Macaroni and Cheese

This dish is simply out of this world. If you have pasta on hand, this fancy meal takes little time to prepare. Whip up a zesty green salad and dinner is done. Use Supreme Pasta (page 172) or Reduced-Carb Pasta (page 174).

PREPARATION TIME: 30 minutes (if you have pasta on hand). BAKING TIME: 25 to 35 minutes.

SERVING SIZE: ⅙ total yield. AMOUNT PER SERVING: 11.7 grams of carb, 28.4 grams of protein. NUMBER OF SERVINGS: 6.

	CHO (g)	PRO (g)
4 cups Supreme Pasta (page 172)	54.7	84.2
½ cup broth or stock (see page 80)	0.5	1.5
1 cup heavy cream	6.4	4.8
2 egg yolks	0.6	2.8
freshly ground black pepper to taste	0	0
salt to taste (about ½ teaspoon)	0	0
5 ounces grated sharp cheddar cheese	2.0	35.5
¾ cup grated Parmesan cheese	3.0	35.7
2 tablespoons butter (¼ stick)	0	0
¼ cup Bread Crumbs I or II (page 25 and page 26)	2.8	5.7
Total	*70.0*	*170.2*

Preheat oven to 325°F or 350°F. Butter a medium-size ovenproof casserole dish or other baking dish.

Cut the pasta in short pieces and put the pieces in a large mixing bowl. Set aside.

Heat the broth and ½ cup cream in a small saucepan. In a small mixing bowl, whisk the egg yolks until smooth. When the broth and cream begin to heat up, add tablespoon amounts to the egg yolks, beating the yolks while you do this. When you have added about ⅓ cup in this way, pour the rest of the liquid into the eggs. Add the remaining cream. Add salt and pepper to this sauce and stir it into the pasta. Add the cheeses to the pasta and stir again. Put the mixture in the casserole dish. Dot with the butter and bread crumbs. Bake for 25 to 35 minutes or until the top begins to brown (do not let the bread crumbs get too dark).

Variation: Lower-Carb Mac and Cheese

Simply use Reduced-Carb Pasta (page 174) instead of Pasta Supreme. The carb count per serving is 8.7 grams; protein is 26.9 grams.

Dumplings/Gnocchi

These amazing little critters can be made quickly. You can cook them in a simmering stock or broth (see page 80), cook them directly in soup, or cook them in water like any other pasta. They can also substitute for potatoes, rice, or whatever.

PREPARATION TIME: 20 to 25 minutes. COOKING TIME: 4 minutes.
SERVING SIZE: 6 dumplings. AMOUNT PER SERVING: 3.9 grams of carb, 7.4 grams of protein. NUMBER OF SERVINGS: 8.

	CHO (g)	PRO (g)
1½ quarts water or stock for cooking dumplings	0	0
⅓ cup cold water	0	0
4 tablespoons (½ stick) cold butter	0	0
⅓ cup stoneground whole-wheat flour	24.1	5.3
¼ cup soy protein powder	0	16.0
¼ cup vital wheat gluten flour	5.6	26.0
salt to taste (about ⅛ teaspoon)	0	0
2 eggs	1.2	12.0
Total	*30.9*	*59.3*

Bring lightly salted water or beef or chicken stock to a simmer and set aside.

In a 1-quart saucepan, heat the cold water and butter until the butter has melted. While the butter is melting, stir together the dry ingredients and mix well.

Once the butter has melted and the water begins to bubble, stir the dry mix all at once into the saucepan. Stir vigorously with a wooden spoon until everything combines into a homogeneous mixture and leaves the sides of the pan (this takes just a few seconds).

Remove the saucepan from the heat and stir in one egg. Stir until the egg is completely absorbed (a wooden spoon works well for this). Add the second egg and repeat the process. The mixture should be soft, like a thick porridge.

Use two teaspoons to drop chunks of the dough about the size of cherries into the simmering water or stock. The dumplings will be

Note: To make the dumplings look more like gnocchi and also more engaging, force the dough into the water through a pastry bag with a ½-inch nozzle. Drop 2-inch segments into the simmering water or stock. If you make the dumplings or gnocchi larger or smaller, just count the total number you end up with and divide by the total count. (The recipe is based on 48 dumplings.)

ready in about 4 minutes; it's okay if some are in the water a little longer. If you want to use dumplings in soup, you can either transfer the cooked dumplings from the water to the soup or cook them directly in the soup.

Serve the dumplings/gnocchi in two ways: Always drain them first and gently pat them dry with paper towels. Put them in a serving bowl and add a little butter to coat them (reheat in the microwave). The other option is to heat a medium-size skillet on medium-low. Add about 2 tablespoons of butter and 1 tablespoon of freshly chopped parsley (in a pinch, use 1 teaspoon dried). When the butter foams (do not brown), add the dumplings/gnocchi and brown them in the butter. It makes them taste and look great.

No-Compromise Thin-Crust Pizza

This pizza crust can hold its own in the company of any thin-crust pizza. It takes 10 minutes to get it in the oven for prebaking. While the crust is in the oven you prepare the toppings. Pile them on the crust and bake a little longer. You can make one 16-inch pizza, or two 10-inchers, or three small ones.

PREPARATION TIME: 20 minutes. TOTAL BAKING TIME: 19 to 33 minutes.
SERVING SIZE: 1 slice. AMOUNT PER SERVING (CRUST ONLY): 5.2 grams of
carb, 4.1 grams of protein. NUMBER OF SERVINGS: 8.

	CHO (g)	PRO (g)
2 tablespoons cold water	0	0
¼ cup hot water	0	0
1 tablespoon olive oil	0	0
1 package rapid-rise yeast	1.2	0
½ cup stoneground whole-wheat flour	36.2	8.0
¼ cup soy protein	0	16.0
2 tablespoons whole almond meal	1.5	3.0
4 tablespoons unprocessed wheat bran	3.0	2.0
salt (about ¼ teaspoon or to taste)	0	0
1 tablespoon soy protein powder (for rolling)	0	4.0
Total	*41.9*	*33.0*

Preheat oven to 425°F. Use a nonstick, heavy-gauge pizza pan.

Combine the cold water, boiling water, and olive oil in a 1-quart mixing bowl. Add the yeast and stir. Wait 5 minutes. Meanwhile, combine all of the other ingredients in a mixing bowl except for the soy protein needed for rolling the dough; stir. Add the dry mixture to the yeast mixture and stir with a fork until the moisture is mostly absorbed. Work the dough by hand until smooth (it takes a few seconds). If the dough is a little too moist, add about 1 teaspoon soy protein powder. Spread some soy protein powder on a large cutting board (put a towel beneath it). Roll out the dough very thin. For example, if you make one 12-inch pizza (not a 16-incher), there will be too much dough. Roll out the dough as if you were making a 16-inch pizza (approximately). Fit the dough on the smaller pan and cut away the overhang. Throw away the extra dough—you will be saving carbs. Do this with any pan or pans you use. Form a small outer edge. Prick the crust bottom many times all over with a fork to prevent bubbles.

Bake the crust for 9 to 11 minutes or until it begins to darken. Build the pizza. For sauce and topping choices see pages 186 and 187. To prevent the edge of the pizza from becoming too dark in the second baking, fold a strip of aluminum foil over it as a guard. Bake the pizza for about 10 to 12 minutes or until nice and bubbly. If you like, you can bake the crust ahead and freeze it (carefully).

Soft-Crust Pizza

If you like soft, chewy pizza, here is a low-carb version that will please you. Soft and thicker crusts require more dough, though, which makes the carb count rise. Make this pizza an occasional treat—perhaps to keep you from running to a pizza parlor or calling for delivery.

Regular pizza dough usually calls for about 3 cups of flour (if you want to make pizza at home). You can make a big pizza with all that flour, but one slice of a 16-inch pizza could have 34.0 grams of carb just for the crust. You can see what you are up against. Regular pizzas are true carb killers. This crust has 7.7 grams of carb per serving.

PREPARATION TIME: 40 minutes. BAKING TIME: 15 to 18 minutes.
SERVING SIZE: 1 slice (12-inch pizza). AMOUNT PER SERVING (CRUST ONLY): 7.7 grams of carb, 7.4 grams of protein. NUMBER OF SERVINGS: 8.

	CHO (g)	PRO (g)
½ cup cold water	0	0
⅓ cup hot water	0	0
4 tablespoons olive oil	0	0
1 package rapid-rise yeast	1.2	0
¾ cup stoneground whole-wheat flour	54.3	15.0
½ cup whole almond meal	6.0	12.0
½ cup soy protein powder	0	32.0
salt (about ¼ teaspoon or to taste)	0	0
Total	*61.5*	*59.0*

Preheat oven to 450°F. Lightly oil a 14-inch pizza pan.

Combine the cold water, boiling water, and olive oil in a medium-size mixing bowl. Add the yeast and stir. While the yeast activates (it needs no added sugar), combine the stoneground whole-wheat flour, almond meal, soy protein powder (except for the last tablespoon), and salt in another mixing bowl; stir. Add the dry mix to the yeast mix and stir with a fork until the moisture is pretty well absorbed. Work the dough by hand until smooth (it takes a few seconds). Cover the bowl and let the dough rise for about 10 minutes.

While the dough rises, prepare sauce and toppings (see pages 186 and 187).

Spread the dough to fit the pizza pan and form an edge. Build the pizza. Bake for about 15 to 18 minutes or until bubbly and done.

Personal Waffle Pizza

(gluten-free)

If you have waffles already made, this becomes almost instant pizza. Even if not, it still is an easy way to make a pizza. And it is gluten-free. While you cook the waffles, you can assemble the toppings and make the sauce. Bake and serve. The best waffles for pizza are, of course, round ones. Figure on using one 7- or 8-inch, circular waffle per person.

PREPARATION TIME: 15 minutes (40 minutes if the waffles must be made).
 BAKING TIME: 10 to 13 minutes.
SERVING SIZE: 1 round 7½-inch waffle (or equivalent). AMOUNT PER SERV-
 ING (WAFFLE ONLY): 4.0 grams of carb, 14.0 grams of protein. NUMBER
 OF SERVINGS: 2.

	CHO (g)	PRO (g)
2 7½-inch Basic Waffles (page 53)	9.6	36.6

If waffles are frozen, remove them from the freezer some hours before they are needed (to ensure that they will be dry). Otherwise, put them briefly in the oven (avoid overbaking). If waffles need to be made, see Basic Waffles on page 53.

Preheat oven to 400°F. Cut out two cardboard circles for each waffle and make them about ½ inch larger than the waffles you are using. Cover the cardboard with aluminum foil. Brush lightly with oil. Put a waffle on top. Set the circles on a cookie sheet. (If your waffle maker cooks only square waffles, use two of them, pushed together, for a serving. Cut cardboard for the size you need.)

Prepare sauce and toppings of your choice (see pages 186 and 187). There is one requirement with waffles that you do not have with a normal pizza crust: waffles made of separate sections may drift apart and are subject to seepage. To prevent this, begin building pizza toppings with a layer of sliced mozzarella or other thinly sliced cheese and put the sauce on top of the cheese. Bake waffles until the toppings are done or nice and bubbly, about 10 to 13 minutes.

Pizza Sauce

This sauce is about as low in carb as you can make it but delivers plenty of zip. You can leave it plain, use the herbs suggested here, or use others you like.

PREPARATION TIME: 5 minutes.

SERVING SIZE: ⅛ total yield. AMOUNT PER SERVING (SAUCE ONLY): 0.8 gram of carb, negligible amount of protein. NUMBER OF SERVINGS: 8.

	CHO (g)	PRO (g)
½ cup canned crushed tomatoes*	6.0	2.0
3 tablespoons olive oil	0	0
2 tablespoons water	0	0
salt to taste (about ½ teaspoon)	0	0
1 teaspoon dried oregano (optional)	0.4	0
2 tablespoons chopped fresh basil (optional)	0.2	0
Total	*6.6*	*2.0*

Mix all ingredients until smooth and spread the sauce evenly over the pizza.

* If you make pizza often, consider freezing crushed tomatoes in ½-cup portions.

Pizza Toppings

Everyone has a favorite way of piling stuff on pizza. Some like it simple; some like it with everything. Here is a pile-everything-on-it idea. Alter the ingredients if you wish, but keep track of the carbs if you make changes.

PREPARATION TIME: 10 minutes.

SERVING SIZE: ⅛ total yield. AMOUNT PER SERVING (TOPPING ONLY): 3.7 grams of carb, 10.3 grams of protein. NUMBER OF SERVINGS: 8.

	CHO (g)	PRO (g)
12 ounces whole-milk mozzarella and cheddar cheese (or other cheese)	7.2	66.0
1 cup chopped green pepper	4.6	0.8
½ cup sliced onion	5.5	0.9
20 sliced canned black olives or 10 fresh cured olives	4.0	0
2 ounces sliced Portobello mushrooms	2.0	1.0
2 ounces pepperoni (about 32 slices)	0	12.0
3 tablespoons freshly chopped basil (or more)	0.3	0
⅔ cup freshly chopped tomatoes*	5.6	1.0
Total	*29.2*	*81.7*

Sauté the mushrooms lightly in a little butter. You can also leave them raw, if you like. Build the layers after you have applied the Pizza Sauce (page 186). You can put the cheese on last or first.

Note: You can easily change pizza toppings. To a base of sauce, add 12 to 16 ounces of the cheese of your choice and any of the following combinations: 3 ounces thinly sliced cured ham, which adds 2.0 grams of protein per pizza slice, ½ cup chopped onion (adds 0.7 grams of carb per pizza slice), 5 ounces smoked salmon (3.3 grams of extra protein per pizza slice). Add salmon for the last 4 minutes of baking. Invent your own toppings.

* Tomatoes that lack flavor make the pizza experience less enjoyable (you are better off using none). Make sure you use ripe, delicious tomatoes. Otherwise, especially in winter, open a can of diced tomatoes and use ½ cup of well-drained little pieces to spread over the pizza instead.

Low-Carb Focaccia (Flatbread)

Whether you call it flatbread or focaccia, it's pretty much the same thing. These breads are from Italy and are baked as flat breads roughly about an inch high from a raised dough. They are given intense flavor with a variety of toppings such as herbs, garlic, onion, cheese, mushrooms, olives, and tomatoes. This bread is great for dipping; it is customarily broken off in pieces rather than cut. There are two flatbread recipes in this section: a raised type and a gluten-free quick bread. Carb and protein counts of the various toppings (see page 187) must be added to the bread. If you were to cut the bread, you would get about 30 pieces that are about 1 by 2 inches (baked in a 9- by 13-inch pan). The larger you make the bread (using bigger pans), the better the carb economy. The breads taste delicious even if you do not make them 1 inch thick. If you do want a thick flatbread, bake the loaves in 12- by 12-inch baking pans and divide the number of pieces by the total carb and protein counts in each recipe.

PREPARATION TIME: 15 minutes. BAKING TIME: 20 minutes.

SERVING SIZE: 1 piece. AMOUNT PER SERVING: 0.8 gram of carb, 4.7 grams of protein. NUMBER OF SERVINGS: 30.

	CHO (g)	PRO (g)
4 ounces cream cheese, soft	3.2	8.4
3 ounces butter (¾ stick), soft	0	0
3 eggs	1.8	18.0
¾ cup soy protein powder	0	48.0
½ cup whey protein powder	6.0	40.0
1 cup whole almond meal	12.0	24.0
1 teaspoon baking powder	1.2	0
salt to taste (about ½ teaspoon or less)	0	0
Total	*24.2*	*138.4*

Preheat oven to 325°F or 350°F. Rub a 9- by 13- by 2-inch (or similar size), nonstick heavy-gauge metal baking pan with olive oil or coconut oil.

Put cream cheese, butter, and one egg in the bowl of an electric mixer and beat with a flat beater until smooth and creamy. Add the remaining eggs and beat briefly again. Add the rest of the ingredients all at once and beat at slow speed just until mixed. Batter will be soft.

Distribute the batter evenly in the pan (use a spatula or knife), but do not make it smooth. Flatbreads are meant to have somewhat rough, uneven tops. Apply the toppings of your choice (pages 190–91). Bake the flatbread for about 20 minutes or until lightly browned.

Raised Focaccia or Flatbread

This is delicious. Try making it into garlic bread (one of the toppings you can apply). If you like, you can double the size of this bread by spreading it out in a 13- by 17-inch pan. It cuts the carbs per piece in half (it doubles the number of pieces), but the pieces will be barely ½ inch thick. If you do this, you need to increase the amount of topping by 50 percent.

PREPARATION TIME: 15 to 20 minutes. BAKING TIME: 18 to 20 minutes.
SERVING SIZE: 1 piece (about 1- by 2- by ¾-inches). AMOUNT PER SERVING: 2.2 grams of carb, 4.1 grams of protein. NUMBER OF SERVINGS: 30.

		CHO (g)	PRO (g)
¾	cup hot water	0	0
4	tablespoons butter (½ stick), soft	0	0
4	tablespoons cold water	0	0
1	package rapid-rise yeast	1.2	0
½	cup stoneground whole-wheat flour	36.2	8.0
1¼	cups whole almond meal	15.0	30.0
½	cup unprocessed wheat bran	6.0	4.0
¾	cup soy protein powder	0	48.0
⅓	cup vital wheat gluten flour	7.5	34.7
	salt to taste (about ¼ teaspoon)	0	0
	Total	*65.9*	*124.7*

Preheat oven to 200°F for 15 minutes and turn off. Lightly butter or oil a 9- by 13-inch nonstick heavy-gauge metal baking pan.

Put the hot water in the bowl of your electric mixer or large food processor (or in a medium-size mixing bowl if you do this by hand). Add the butter and stir until dissolved. Add the cold water and yeast and stir. Wait 5 minutes.

Put the dry ingredients, including the salt, in a mixing bowl and mix well. Add this mixture to the yeast mixture. Use a dough hook to knead the dough in the mixer for about 5 minutes. (If you do not have a dough hook, use a flat beater; this is not as large an amount of dough as used for making bread.) If working manually, stir the dry mixture with a fork into the yeast mixture. Take over by hand and knead the dough for 5 minutes. (If needed, rub a little soy protein powder on your palm, although this dough is not sticky.)

Press the dough flat into the baking pan and try to get it level, but do not strive for a smooth surface. Apply toppings of your choice (pages 190–91). Bake the flatbread for about 18 to 20 minutes or until lightly browned.

Focaccia (Flatbread) Topping I

SERVING SIZE: Topping for 1 piece (about 1 by 2 inches). AMOUNT PER SERVING: 0.4 gram of carb, negligible amount of protein. NUMBER OF SERVINGS: 30. PREPARATION TIME: 5 to 10 minutes.

		CHO (g)	PRO (g)
2	teaspoons olive oil	0	0
1	tablespoon dried rosemary	0.7	0
12	fresh brined Kalamata olives, sliced	5.0	0
1	teaspoon garlic powder	2.3	0.5
3	teaspoons dried minced onions	3.4	0.6
	Total	*11.4*	*1.1*

Brush a film of olive oil gently and evenly over the soft batter. Sprinkle the rest of the ingredients evenly over the top. Bake as directed.

Focaccia (Flatbread) Topping II

SERVING SIZE: Topping for 1 piece (about 1 by 2 inches). AMOUNT PER SERVING: 0.5 gram of carb, 0.8 gram of protein. NUMBER OF SERVINGS: 30. PREPARATION TIME: 5–10 minutes.

	CHO (g)	PRO (g)
2 teaspoons olive oil	0	0
½ cup chopped sun-dried tomatoes packed in oil	8.0	4.0
1 teaspoon dried minced onions	1.7	0
¾ cup shredded mozzarella (or cheese of choice)	2.1	18.6
½ teaspoon garlic powder	1.8	0
3 tablespoons freshly chopped basil	0.4	0
1 teaspoon dried oregano	0.5	0
½ tablespoon olive oil (optional)	0	0
Total	*14.5*	*22.6*

Brush the olive oil gently and evenly over the batter. Lightly top the batter with the ingredients and finish with a drizzle of olive oil (optional). Bake as directed.

Focaccia (Flatbread) Topping III (Garlic Bread)

SERVING SIZE: Topping for 1 piece (about 1 by 2 inches). AMOUNT PER SERVING: 0.5 gram of carb, 1.3 grams of protein. NUMBER OF SERVINGS: 30. PREPARATION TIME: 5 minutes.

	CHO (g)	PRO (g)
2 teaspoons olive oil	0	0
2 tablespoons butter, soft (¼ stick)	0	0
5 teaspoons garlic powder (or 10 to 12 crushed cloves)	11.5	2.5
¾ cup grated Parmesan cheese	3.0	35.7
Total	*14.5*	*38.2*

Brush a film of olive oil evenly and gently over the soft dough. Add a layer of soft butter.

Sprinkle the garlic powder or crushed garlic over the flatbread. Sprinkle cheese over garlic. Bake as directed.

LOW-CARB TORTILLAS, TORTILLA CHIPS, AND TACOS

The sky-high carb count in almost all Mexican foods generally takes them off the table for low-carb dieters.* So you have to pitch in and make your own. If you can spare the time—and if you love tortillas—you won't regret it. The tortillas come in a range of carb counts. No tortilla exceeds 6.0 grams of carb.

Tortillas need to be rolled out; a standard tortilla press will not work with this dough. Still, this dough will roll over for you nicely, with nary a pitfall. You can make corn tortillas, flour tortillas, and gluten-free low-carb tortillas. Tortillas are easily turned into chips (and they are not fried, unlike commercial chips, but are every bit as good). Add some spices and you get spicy chips. Bake chips smothered with cheese and you have nachos. Tacos can be an absolute pain to make—you have to hold the taco with your fingers in the hot fat and guide it into its crisply fried, taco U-shape. There's the potential for burning and it takes time to do. However, you can buy a taco rack that makes the job easy. You simply drape tacos over the rack and bake them into shape. (If you cannot find one, see "Mail Order Sources.") With so many different tortilla recipes and the many chips you can make, the Mexican world will open up to you—again.

---

* An exception is a low-carb tortilla made by La Tortilla Factory in Santa Rosa and widely available in supermarkets. Try them and compare.

Corn Tortillas

Made with masa harina, these tortillas have some of that wonderful corn flavor but far fewer carb grams. You have to roll them out. Still, it is really easy to do; you don't have to have an expert touch for the job. Try this and you will be sold on making them and eating them.

PREPARATION TIME: 25 to 30 minutes. COOKING TIME: 3 minutes.
SERVING SIZE: 1 tortilla. AMOUNT PER SERVING: 5.4 grams of carb, 8.0 grams
  of protein. NUMBER OF SERVINGS: 9.

	CHO (g)	PRO (g)
¼ cup hot water	0	0
3 tablespoons butter (1.5 oz), soft	0	0
2 tablespoons cold water	0	0
3 tablespoons olive oil	0	0
½ cup masa harina (enriched corn flour)	38.0	8.0
¼ cup vital wheat gluten flour	5.6	26.0
⅓ cup soy protein powder	0	21.5
3 tablespoons unprocessed wheat bran	2.1	1.9
¼ cup whole almond meal	3.0	6.0
salt (a few shakes)	0	0
2 tablespoons soy protein powder (for rolling dough)	0	8.0
Total	*48.7*	*71.4*

In a small or medium-size mixing bowl, mix the hot water with the butter; stir to dissolve. Add the cold water and the oil. Set aside.

In another mixing bowl, combine all of the dry ingredients except for the soy protein powder needed for rolling out the dough. Add the dry mixture to the liquid mixture and stir until the liquid is absorbed. Take over by hand and work into a fairly soft dough that can be rolled out. If more moisture is needed (it should rarely be necessary), add cold water by the teaspoon. If the dough is too soft, it will not roll out easily. If this happens, correct it by adding a teaspoon of soy protein powder or as needed. Divide the dough in nine equal chunks about the size of small plums; cover.

If you have a tortilla press, press chunks of dough in one to form the tortillas.

To roll out tortillas, sprinkle a little soy protein powder (about 1 teaspoon) on a large, heavy cutting board (approximately 14 by 19 inches). Put a kitchen towel under it to keep the board from sliding. Roll a piece of the dough lightly in the soy protein powder and flatten it with your fingers into a circle about 3 or 4 inches in diameter. Continue with a rolling pin. Strive to make circular shapes (this becomes easier with practice). Make the tortillas about 7 inches in diameter; they shrink about an inch when cooked. If the shape becomes too irregular, control the circle by sculpting with a knife. You can also put a sharp-edged lid or flan on the tortilla and press down to get a perfect shape. Save all the dough you cut away—it will help form the last tortilla.

Finish rolling out the tortillas. When you come to the last one or two, heat a griddle on medium-low. Cook each tortilla on the dry griddle for about 10 seconds on each side. Put them on a cooling rack. If you do not want to use the tortillas right away, cool them completely and keep them in an airtight plastic bag. They keep for about a week in the fridge; otherwise, freeze. If you want to warm a tortilla to fill, heat it between paper towels in a microwave.

Variation: Lower-Carb Tortillas

You can reduce carb grams if you cut the masa harina in half and double the amount of soy protein powder. It will reduce each tortilla to 3.3 grams of carb and increase protein to 9.3 grams.

Flour Tortillas

Made with stoneground whole-wheat flour, these tortillas are still relatively low in carb. It is really easy to make them. Follow the directions for making Corn Tortillas on page 193.

PREPARATION TIME: 25 to 30 minutes. COOKING TIME: 3 minutes.
SERVING SIZE: 1 tortilla. AMOUNT PER SERVING: 5.0 grams of carb, 5.3 grams
   of protein. NUMBER OF SERVINGS: 9.

	CHO (g)	PRO (g)
¼ cup hot water	0	0
2 tablespoons butter, soft (¼ stick)	0	0
3 tablespoons cold water	0	0
2 tablespoons olive oil	0	0
⅔ cup stoneground whole-wheat flour	36.2	8.0
⅓ cup soy protein powder	0	21.3
¼ cup unprocessed wheat bran	3.0	2.0
¼ cup whole almond meal	3.0	6.0
salt (a few shakes)	0	0
2 tablespoons soy protein powder (for rolling dough)	0	8.0
Total	*42.2*	*45.3*

Gluten-Free Tortillas

Low-carb and gluten-free tortillas—a great combination. By the time you load these tortillas with goodies, you might be hard-pressed to tell that they lack the flour that is part of the other tortillas in this book. Even if you usually use gluten flour, it is well worth giving these tortillas a try because they are so very low in carbs—under 3.0 grams per tortilla. Follow the directions for making Corn Tortillas on page 193.

PREPARATION TIME: 25 to 30 minutes. COOKING TIME: 3 minutes.
SERVING SIZE: 1 tortilla. AMOUNT PER SERVING: 2.8 grams of carb, 16.3 grams of protein. NUMBER OF SERVINGS: 7 to 8.

		CHO (g)	PRO (g)
¼	cup hot water	0	0
2	tablespoons butter (¼ stick), soft	0	0
3	tablespoons cold water	0	0
2	tablespoons olive oil	0	0
¼	cup whey protein powder	3.0	20.0
¾	cup soy protein powder	0	48.0
1¼	cups whole almond meal	15.0	30.0
	salt (a few shakes)	0	0
4	tablespoons soy protein powder (for rolling dough)	0	16.0
	Total	*18.0*	*114.0*

Variation: Low-Carb Tacos

Use any tortilla recipe of your choice. Follow the directions for making the dough as given for Corn Tortillas on page 193, but when you roll out the tortillas, make them about 4½ inches in diameter or the size you need to fit them over your taco rack. The shells should drape completely over the rack but not curl at the bottom. They will still shrink as they bake and dry. Preheat the oven to 350°F. Bake the tacos for about 10 minutes or until crisp. Unless you can find a taco rack that holds more than three or four tacos at a time, you might want to buy a set of two racks if you prefer to make a larger batch and cut down on total baking time (see "Mail Order Sources").

Low-Carb Chips

Chips can be made from any tortilla dough. You can make them from any of the tortilla recipes: Corn Tortillas (page 193), Flour Tortillas (page 195), or Gluten-Free Tortillas (page 196), including the reduced-carb versions. You just roll out the dough and cut the chips into the size you want. The only recipe spelled out for chips, spicy or plain, is for chips made from Corn Tortillas. The directions apply to whichever tortilla recipe you choose. The spicy chips tend to roll out a little less easily than the plain chips; it is best to use smaller portions of dough than you would for the plain chips.

Spicy Corn Chips

Crunchy, delicious, low-carb—and not drenched in fat. The dough needs to be rolled out and cut into chips. It is fairly easy to do but takes a little time. The results are highly rewarding. This recipe makes relatively mild chips; increase the spices to suit your taste.

PREPARATION TIME: 30 to 40 minutes to mix and roll out dough. BAKING TIME: 10 to 12 minutes per batch.

SERVING SIZE: 1 ounce of tortilla chips (about 12 to 14 pieces 1 by 1½ inches). AMOUNT PER SERVING: 9.6 grams of carb, 9.2 grams of protein. NUMBER OF SERVINGS: 7 or 8.

	CHO (g)	PRO (g)
¼ cup hot water	0	0
3 tablespoons butter, soft	0	0
2 tablespoons cold water	0	0
3 tablespoons olive oil	0	0
½ cup masa harina (enriched corn flour)	38.0	8.0
¼ cup vital wheat gluten flour	5.6	26.0
⅓ cup soy protein powder	0	16.0
3 tablespoons unprocessed wheat bran	2.3	1.5
¼ cup whole almond meal	3.0	6.0
1 tablespoon ground chili powder (or as desired)	1.5	0.9
1 teaspoon garlic powder	2.3	0.5
½ teaspoon cumin (optional)	0.4	0
cayenne pepper (dash or as desired)	0	0
salt to taste (a few shakes or as desired)	0	0
freshly ground black pepper (as desired)	0	0
2 tablespoons soy protein powder (for rolling dough)	0	8.0
Total	*53.1*	*66.9*

In a small or medium-size mixing bowl, mix the hot water with the butter, stir to dissolve. Add the cold water and olive oil.

In another mixing bowl, combine all of the dry ingredients except for the soy protein powder needed for rolling. Mix well. Add the dry mixture to the liquid mixture and stir with a fork until the liquid is absorbed. Use your hands to shape the dough into a smooth ball. Cover. Chill for about 1 hour or longer.

When you are ready to proceed, preheat oven to 350°F.

Sprinkle a tiny bit of soy protein powder on a large cutting board. Pinch off a chunk of dough about the size of a large walnut. Roll it in the soy protein powder and flatten it lightly with your hand, shaping it into a rectangle. Roll the piece as thin as you can make it. Divide the dough into three or four equal pieces and stack them. Cut strips of about 1 inch by 1½ inches or make the chips any size you want them. They will shrink by about one-third when they bake. Put chips on two large, nonstick, heavy-gauge metal cookie sheets (remember, they will shrink, not expand). Bake them for 10 to 12 minutes or until lightly browned. Slide onto a rack to cool and to dry them completely.

Variation: **Plain Corn Chips**

To make plain chips, follow the recipe for Spicy Corn Chips on page 197. Leave out the spices but retain the salt and pepper. This saves a total of 6.8 grams of carb in the recipe; 1 ounce of chips has 4.8 grams of carb.

Variation: **Nachos**

These cheese-flavored chips can be made from Spicy Corn Chips (page 197) or Plain Corn Chips (above). Preheat oven to 350°F. Put cooked chips on cookie sheet. (This takes about one-half recipe of chips.) Sprinkle about ¾ cup grated cheddar cheese over the chips. Bake in oven until the cheese has melted (about 6 to 10 minutes). This adds about 3.0 grams of protein to each serving (1 ounce) of Spicy Corn Chips and has no effect on carb counts.

Variation: **Reduced-Carb Spicy Corn Chips**

You can save some carb grams and still get very tasty chips. Follow the recipe for Spicy Corn Chips on page 197, but reduce masa harina (corn flour) to ¼ cup and increase soy protein powder to ½ cup. The yield will be the same. An ounce of chips has 4.2 grams of carb and 11.4 grams of protein. You can also make Plain Corn Chips (above), which saves another 0.7 grams of carb per 1 ounce serving.

World's Best Guacamole

*If you're a guac lover, this recipe will become a staple in your reper-
toire. If you've got the ingredients on hand, you can whip up a
delicious bowlful in minutes to serve with Reduced-Carb Spicy Corn
Chips (page 198) or over lettuce as a salad with Mexican dishes.
Although this recipe makes a smallish batch, it can be multiplied
easily to feed a whole hoard.*

PREPARATION TIME: 15 minutes.
SERVING SIZE: ½ cup. AMOUNT PER SERVING: 7.9 grams of carb, 4.4 grams of
protein. NUMBER OF SERVINGS: 4.

	CHO (g)	PRO (g)
½ cup chopped red onion	3.8	0.6
2 tablespoons plus 1 teaspoon lemon or lime juice	2.7	0.1
1 clove garlic, minced or pressed	0.9	0.2
4 ripe Haas avocados, peeled and chopped (toss with lemon juice to prevent browning)	19.2	15.9
1 tomato, seeded and diced	4.4	1.1
2 tablespoons freshly chopped cilantro	0.1	0.1
1 Serrano pepper, seeded and minced	0.2	0.1
½ teaspoon salt	0	0
½ teaspoon black pepper	0.4	0.1
Total	*31.7*	*18.2*

Soak the chopped onion in a small bowl of water plus 1 teaspoon
of lemon or lime juice to take the strength of the onion bite away.
Trim cilantro and mince finely. Trim and seed the Serrano pepper;
mince finely. Always wash your hands immediately after working
with fresh hot chile peppers, as the residual pepper oils can burn or
blister the skin or eyes.

Put 2 tablespoons lemon or lime juice into the bowl you'll use for
the guacamole. Add the garlic to the lemon or lime juice in the bowl.

Mash the chopped avocado thoroughly with a fork or potato masher
—the resultant mixture should be smooth and relatively lump-free.

Drain the citrus water from the onions and add them to the mashed
avocado. Add the tomato, cilantro, and Serrano pepper, as well as the
salt and pepper. Fold all of the ingredients together to mix well.

Serve immediately, if possible. To store for up to 1 day in the refrigerator, press a square of plastic wrap directly onto the surface of the
guacamole in the bowl, leaving no room for air; take the plastic wrap
right up the inner sides of the bowl. Cover the bowl tightly with a lid or
with more plastic wrap. Air is the enemy of the delicate oils in an avocado and will turn it an unappealing gray-brown given the opportunity.

Chile Con Queso (Spicy Cheese Dip)

This easy variation on the Tex-Mex classic is made with good-quality cheeses (instead of processed ones) and fresh ingredients. Thinned slightly, you can use it as a cheese sauce for enchiladas or even over chicken breasts. This version is moderately spicy, but you can alter the heat to your taste by varying the amount of powdered hot chili pepper you add. Like it hotter? Crank it up with some crushed dried red chile peppers or with a bit of habañero chile! The recipe doesn't keep more than a few hours without losing its creaminess, so we've presented about 2 cups here; however, it can be multiplied easily for larger gatherings. Eat it freshly made, if possible.

PREPARATION TIME: 10 minutes. COOKING TIME: 5 minutes.
SERVING SIZE: ½ cup. AMOUNT PER SERVING: 2.9 grams of carb, 12.2 grams of protein. NUMBER OF SERVINGS: 4.

	CHO (g)	PRO (g)
5 ounces white cheddar cheese	4.5	35.5
2 ounces mozzarella cheese	1.2	11.0
¼ cup heavy cream	1.6	1.3
¾ cup chicken broth (see page 80)	1.1	1.1
2 tablespoons seeded and diced tomatoes	0.8	0
2 tablespoons canned roasted and peeled mild green chile	2.0	0
¼ teaspoon cumin	0.2	0
1 pinch hot chili powder or cayenne pepper	0	0
2 teaspoons freshly chopped cilantro	0	0
Total	*11.4*	*48.9*

Place all of the ingredients in a medium-size saucepan and cook over medium-low heat, stirring constantly, until the cheeses have melted and the consistency is uniform and smooth.

Alternatively, you can cook in a microwave oven in a covered microwave-safe dish. Heat on high for 2 minutes, stir, then heat again in 1-minute increments, stirring between each, until the cheeses have completely melted and the consistency is smooth.

To make a cheese sauce, thin with chicken broth, adding only an ounce at a time, stirring between additions.

Salsa Roja (Red Sauce)

When the occasion takes you south of the border, a roasted poblano pepper and tomato salsa will hit the spot. Perfect for dipping Reduced-Carb Spicy Corn Chips (page 198), adding to Quesadillas (page 206), or spicing up enchiladas, tacos, or nachos made the low-carb way. The recipe can be multiplied easily for big crowds.

PREPARATION TIME: 20 minutes. COOKING TIME: 5 minutes.
SERVING SIZE: 1/16 total yield. AMOUNT PER SERVING: 4.5 grams of carb, negligible amount of protein. NUMBER OF SERVINGS: 16.

		CHO (g)	PRO (g)
ROASTING INGREDIENTS			
1	poblano chile pepper, sliced	3.6	0.9
1/2	cup chopped red onion	3.8	0.6
2	cloves garlic, peeled	1.8	0
1	tablespoon peanut oil	0	0
RAW INGREDIENTS			
1/4	cup chopped red onion	1.9	0
2	whole Roma tomatoes	4.4	1.1
2	tablespoons freshly chopped cilantro	0.1	0
1	tablespoon black pepper	0.8	2.6
14	ounces canned Fire Roasted tomatoes, drained and diced	24.0	4.0
1/2	ounce lime juice (about 1 lime)	1.4	0
1/2	ounce lemon juice (about 1/2 lemon)	1.3	0
FOR BLENDING			
14	ounces canned Fire Roasted tomatoes, drained and diced	24.0	4.0
1	canned chipotle pepper*	2.8	0.7
12	ounces water	0	0
	Total	*69.9*	*13.9*

Heat a griddle on medium and roast the onion, garlic, and poblano pepper in the peanut oil. Once darkened, remove from the griddle and cool slightly. Set aside.

In a blender or food processor, blend the ingredients for blending, pulse to combine, then add the roasted ingredients and blend to a chunky texture.

Stir in the raw ingredients by hand. Refrigerate, tightly covered, until serving time.

---

* If you like, you may substitute 1 teaspoon of hickory smoke liquid and 1/4 teaspoon of cayenne pepper for the chipotle.

Salsa Verde (Green Sauce)

Ideal for dipping with low-carb tortilla chips but delicious with chicken enchiladas or quesadillas (low-carb, of course), this fresh green salsa will soon become one of your favorite Mexican condiments. This recipe makes a quart, which will keep in the refrigerator for several days if tightly sealed, but can easily be made in larger batches for bigger groups.

PREPARATION TIME: 30 minutes. COOKING TIME: 5 to 10 minutes.
SERVING SIZE: ¹⁄₁₆ total yield. AMOUNT PER SERVING: 2.5 grams of carb, negligible amount of protein. NUMBER OF SERVINGS: 16.

		CHO (g)	PRO (g)
1	tablespoon peanut oil	0	0
1½	pounds whole green tomatillos	26.8	6.5
¼	cup chopped red onion	1.9	0
1	Serrano pepper	0.2	0
2	cloves garlic	1.8	0
2	teaspoons black pepper	1.8	0.6
½	ounce lemon juice (about ½ lemon)	1.3	0
½	ounce lime juice (about ½ lime)	1.4	0
1	tablespoon salt	0	0
10	ounces water	0	0
2	tablespoons freshly chopped cilantro	0.1	0
1	ripe Haas avocado, peeled and chopped	4.8	4.0
1	lime, cut into wedges	0	0
	Total	*40.1*	*11.1*

Heat peanut oil on a griddle or in a large skillet, then roast the tomatillos, onion, Serrano pepper, and garlic until they begin to brown. Cover them with ice in a bowl to cool. When cool enough to handle, remove husks from the tomatillos and discard.

Blend the roasted ingredients with the next five ingredients and refrigerate, tightly covered, for up to 2 days.

Just before serving, add the cilantro to the blended ingredients and pulse a few times in a blender or food processor to lightly blend. You should still see small pieces of cilantro leaves in the salsa. Add the avocado and again pulse a few times, leaving some chunks of avocado intact.

Pour into a serving bowl and garnish with lime wedges and fresh cilantro leaves.

Muy Bueno Refried Black Soybeans

When a real Mexican fiesta is what you crave, what's a soft taco, fajita, or enchilada without the refried beans? Now you can have it all! Or if you're in the mood for a party snack, the refried recipe makes a great bean dip that's high in protein, low in carbs, and long on comfort.

PREPARATION TIME: 20 minutes. COOKING TIME: 5 minutes.
SERVING SIZE: ½ cup. AMOUNT PER SERVING: 3.1 grams of carb, 6.3 grams of protein. NUMBER OF SERVINGS: 8.

		CHO (g)	PRO (g)
2	cans (15 ounces each) organic black soybeans rinsed, drained, and mashed	22.4	48.4
5	ounces chicken broth	0.6	1.9
2	tablespoons coconut oil	0	0
2	tablespoons chopped red onion	1.4	0
½	teaspoon salt (or to taste)	0	0
½	teaspoon black pepper	0.5	0
	Total	*24.9*	*50.3*

In a blender or food processor, puree the black soybeans and chicken broth until the consistency is relatively smooth.

In a medium-size saucepan, heat the coconut oil on medium or medium-low heat and sauté the onion in the oil until just beginning to turn golden—do not brown or burn.

Carefully add the bean puree to the saucepan—it may pop a bit, so watch out! Heat the beans. Stir in the salt and pepper. Keep warm until serving time (or reheat on stovetop). You may wish to stir in a bit more chicken broth if the beans become too stiff.

Variation: Black Soybean Dip

You'll simply need to add another ½ cup or so of chicken broth to make a thinner mixture, ½ teaspoon cumin powder, and a dash of hot red chile powder (if desired) for zip and an insignificant increase in carbs per serving. Serve with Reduced-Carb Spicy Corn Chips (page 198) or other chips of your choice.

Bean and Cheese Burritos

Have you got the refried soybeans and tortillas? If you do, you are about to put a scrumptious meal together in just a few minutes. Two makes a meal and one makes a marvelous low-carb snack.

PREPARATION TIME: 10 minutes. COOKING TIME: 30–45 seconds.

SERVING SIZE: 2 burritos. AMOUNT PER SERVING: 14.7 grams of carb, 36.5 grams of protein. NUMBER OF SERVINGS: 2.

		CHO (g)	PRO (g)
4	Corn Tortillas (page 193)	21.6	32.0
1	cup Refried Black Soybeans (page 203)	6.2	12.6
1	cup shredded cheddar or jack cheese	1.6	28.4
	salt to taste	0	0
	freshly ground black pepper to taste	0	0
	Total	*29.4*	*73.0*

If needed, soften tortillas in microwave (between paper towels) for a second. Put ¼ cup refried beans on each tortilla; top with ¼ cup shredded cheese. Roll up tortillas and put them in a microwave-safe tray. Heat briefly on high until they are hot and the cheese has melted.

You can also use the Spicy Cheese Dip on page 200.

Green Enchiladas

If you have some tortillas sitting in the fridge, you can make green enchiladas in an impressive hurry. What is nice is that it is not much more work to make smaller or larger batches. This recipe is for three, but the high-carb count means maintenance-suitable only. Enjoy just one at other times along with a pork chop or chicken breast. Adjust it as you like. You must vary the carb content for the tortillas if you are not using the Corn Tortillas (page 193).

These enchiladas don't contain meat. You can easily add an ounce of either cooked and shredded beef or chicken to each tortilla. (It will raise the protein count per serving to approximately 37.0 grams.)

PREPARATION TIME: 25 to 30 minutes. BAKING TIME: 8 to 10 minutes.
SERVING SIZE: 2 enchiladas. AMOUNT PER SERVING: 19.3 grams of carb, 26.0 grams of protein. NUMBER OF SERVINGS: 3.

	CHO (g)	PRO (g)
⅔ cup chopped onion	5.5	0.9
6 Corn Tortillas (page 193)	32.5	47.6
1 tablespoon olive oil	0	0
4 ounces shredded Mexican Four Cheeses	0.8	26.0
½ cup canned and drained diced green chili pepper	4.0	0
1 cup canned green chili enchilada sauce	12.0	2.0
½ cup sour cream	3.2	1.6
2 tablespoons freshly chopped cilantro	0	0
Total	*58.0*	*78.1*

Preheat oven to 350°F. Butter or oil a 9- by 13-inch glass baking dish.

Heat oil in a small skillet on medium heat. Add the onion and cook until limp and transparent. Remove from the skillet and set aside.

If the tortillas are a little stiff, warm them for a few seconds between paper towels in a microwave. Lay them out to add the filling. Divide the onion, 2 ounces of cheese, and pepper among the tortillas. Fold them over and put seam-side down in the baking dish. Pour the green sauce over the enchiladas. Sprinkle with the remaining 2 ounces of cheese. Bake for about 8 to 10 minutes or until bubbly. Garnish with the sour cream and cilantro and serve.

Quesadillas

What quesadillas all share in common is cheese, but there are several wondrous ways of getting this cheese into or onto them. They can be cooked along the lines of pizza. Pile cheese on a tortilla (perhaps also some additional toppings) and bake the quesadilla in the oven (on a cookie sheet) or simply grill it on an ungreased griddle or skillet until crisp, lightly browned, and the cheese bubbles. Another option is to get a layered look by putting a lid on top of the filling with a second tortilla. Layered tortillas can be heated and cooked until browned and crisp on both sides in the oven or on a griddle (you need to flip them if you use a griddle). Put them in a microwave until the cheese melts (these quesadillas will be soft). Finally, tortillas can be folded over like an omelet and stuffed with cheese and whatever you like. Bake them in the oven or cook them in a skillet (turn once). Whichever way you choose, it takes only a few minutes and just seconds in the microwave.

You can use any topping in addition to the basic one—cheese. Choose jack, cheddar, or mixes. (As a rule of thumb, use about ¼ to ⅓ cup of cheese for one quesadilla.) You can add chopped olives, chopped green onions, chopped peppers, chopped tomatoes, sliced mushrooms, even thinly sliced ham, chicken, or ground beef. Look around your fridge: just about anything goes. Garnish the quesadillas with sour cream, salsa, and guacamole. Make a list of what you are using and keep track of both the carbs and the protein.

Pasta "Arroz Verde"

You will be surprised how good this imitation rice really tastes. So it isn't rice, but it is real pasta. By the time you fry it and add delicious spices and other flavoring, you will love it. It goes well with a lot of Mexican food—from enchiladas to refried beans. This recipe is based on Pasta "Fried Rice" which appears on page 176; however, since it has been changed to a Mexican version, the recipe is repeated here with the variations.

PREPARATION TIME: 25 minutes (add 30 minutes or 1 hour if you have to make the pasta). COOKING TIME: 15 minutes.

SERVING SIZE: 1 cup. AMOUNT PER SERVING: 9.8 grams of carb, 23.5 grams of protein. NUMBER OF SERVINGS: 5.

		CHO (g)	PRO (g)
4	cups Reduced-Carb Pasta (page 174)	30.4	89.6
2	poblano chiles (roasted, peeled, cleaned, seeded*	4.0	0
2	tablespoons peanut oil	0	0
4	eggs	2.4	24.0
1	cup chopped scallion (green and white parts)	4.8	1.8
1	Serrano pepper, seeded and minced	0.1	0
1	cup chopped green pepper	4.6	0
2	cloves garlic, minced (or ½ teaspoon garlic powder)	1.8	0
¼	cup freshly chopped cilantro or parsley	0.5	0.5
½	cup broth (see page 80) or more if needed	0.5	1.5
	salt to taste	0	0
2	tablespoons butter (¼ stick) (optional)	0	0
	Total	*49.1*	*117.4*

On a large cutting board, cut the pasta into pieces approximately ½ to 1 inch long. A mezzaluna works well for this.

Heat a large, heavy skillet on medium-low. Add 1 tablespoon peanut oil.

Lightly beat the eggs. Pour them in the hot peanut oil and allow to spread as you would for an omelet. Do not stir. As soon as the eggs

---

* If you cannot find poblano chiles use, instead, one large, mild green chile and treat the same way.

are cooked on one side and show dryness on top (it takes about a minute), turn the whole sheet of eggs with a spatula and cook for about 30 seconds on the other side. Spread a double layer of paper towels on a large cutting board and put the eggs on it. Allow to cool for handling. Remove the paper towels and roll the sheet of eggs as if it were a jelly roll. Cut into thin strips, then cut the other way, so that the pieces are approximately 1 by ½ inch long (it's okay if you want to make them larger).

Add 1 tablespoon peanut oil to the skillet. Sauté the chopped scallion for about 2 minutes. Add the minced Serrano pepper, green pepper, garlic, and cilantro. Cook for about 1 minute. Add the chopped pasta and heat through, stirring all the time, to allow the pasta to absorb the flavors from the skillet. Add the broth as needed to keep the "rice" moist. Add the eggs last and stir again until the meal is hot. Season with salt. Add butter, if desired. Stir and serve.

7

LOW-CARB COMFORT FOOD
VEGGIES AND SIDE DISHES

When people adopt a low-carb lifestyle, they usually enjoy digging into roasted meats, fish with buttery sauces, and the crispy skin of a baked chicken—particularly if they're newly recruited from the ranks of the low-fat, high-carb crowd. But after the newness wears off, the question invariably arises: What do I put on my plate in place of potatoes, peas, rice, corn, and beans? In the past, the options ran mainly toward the green—salads, green beans, broccoli, and the like—fueling the constant counterpoint of the low-carb hecklers that such a diet is devoid of a variety of fruits and vegetables.

The *Protein Power LifePlan* disabused the dieting public of the notion that low-carb meant a dearth of color on the plate, reminding us of the wide range of choices that can easily be a part of an insulin-controlling lower carbohydrate approach to nutrition. There's no reason not to add tomatoes, red, yellow, and green peppers, summer and winter squashes, mushrooms, onions, garlic, and a host of others to the spinach, broccoli, cauliflower, cabbage, green beans, zucchini, and asparagus of yore.

You'll find dozens of unusual and tasty methods for preparing delicious vegetable side dishes, including some you thought you'd never see again on a low-carb plate: Zucchini Fritters and Breaded Eggplant Fritters. Plus, we've given you some low-carb imposters such as Mock Mashed Potatoes that you'll be hard-pressed to tell from the real thing—in fact, some people even like them better! You be the judge.

Baked Black Soybeans

These yummy baked beans take 10 minutes to throw together. They need to bake for a few hours, but they're worth it. Even if you do not need that many, you might freeze some. Otherwise, just cut the recipe in half. These beans taste even better the next day. They freeze well, too.

PREPARATION TIME: 10 minutes. BAKING TIME: 3 hours.
SERVING SIZE: 1 cup. AMOUNT PER SERVING: 8.7 grams of carb, 12.9 grams of
  protein. NUMBER OF SERVINGS: 5.

		CHO (g)	PRO (g)
3	slices of thick bacon	0	9.0
2	cans (15 ounces each) black soybeans, drained and rinsed	22.4	48.4
½	cup chopped onion (or 1½ teaspoons dried)	5.5	0.9
2	teaspoons hickory smoke liquid	6.0	0
2	teaspoons Dijon-type mustard	0.5	0.5
1	tablespoon tomato paste	2.5	1.0
	salt to taste (about ½ teaspoon)	0	0
	freshly ground black pepper to taste	0	0
2	teaspoons Worcestershire sauce	1.0	0
4	packets Splenda sugar substitute (or to taste)	4.0	0
1½	cups stock or broth (see page 80)	1.5	4.5
4	tablespoons butter (½ stick)	0	0
	Total	*43.4*	*64.3*

Preheat oven to 300°F; butter or oil a medium-size ovenproof casserole dish. Cut the bacon in small pieces; cook in a heavy skillet until done. Drain the cooked bacon thoroughly on the paper towels.

Mix all of the ingredients except the butter into a smooth sauce.

Put the soybean mixture in the casserole and stir. Dot with the butter. Cover and bake for 3 hours. Adjust seasoning and serve.

Vegetarian Chili with Black Soybeans

You can have this meal on the table in about an hour. Serve with sour cream, shredded cheddar or jack cheese, and, of course, Spicy Corn Chips (page 191).

PREPARATION TIME: 10 minutes. COOKING TIME: 1 hour.
SERVING SIZE: ¾ cup. AMOUNT PER SERVING: 8.9 grams of carb, 8.3 grams of protein. NUMBER OF SERVINGS: 4.

		CHO (g)	PRO (g)
15	ounces canned black soybeans, drained and rinsed	11.2	24.2
2	tablespoons olive oil or coconut oil	0	0
2	tablespoons butter (¼ stick)	0	0
½	cup chopped onion (or 2 teaspoons dried)	5.5	0.9
2	tablespoons chili powder	3.0	1.8
1	teaspoon dried oregano	0.5	0
1¼	cups canned crushed tomatoes	15.0	5.0
½	cup stock or broth (see page 80)	0.5	1.5
	salt to taste (about ½ teaspoon)	0	0
	freshly ground black pepper to taste	0	0
4	tablespoons butter (½ stick)	0	0
	Total	*35.7*	*33.4*

Heat a small skillet on medium-low. Add the oil and butter. When the butter bubbles (do not brown), sauté the onion until soft. Turn heat to low and add the chili powder and oregano. Stir for about 2 minutes. Add the beans and stir. Add all of the other ingredients and simmer the chili slowly, covered, for about 1 hour, stirring occasionally. Adjust seasonings and serve.

Vegetarian Burgers

These burgers or bean cakes take barely 10 minutes to put together and are sure to be a big hit anytime. They are a good potato and rice substitute. Make them for breakfast with a side of fruit and cottage cheese. Make them in place of hash browns. They taste much better than the vegetarian patties you can buy in the supermarket. Have them on a burger-size Magic Roll (page 22). You can make the burger mix at night and form the patties in the morning. You can also freeze these burgers and thaw them in the microwave.

PREPARATION TIME: 10 minutes. COOKING TIME: 6 to 8 minutes.

SERVING SIZE: 2 cakes. AMOUNT PER SERVING: 6.5 grams of carb, 8.8 grams of protein. NUMBER OF SERVINGS: 4 to 5.

		CHO (g)	PRO (g)
15	ounces black soybeans, drained and mashed	11.2	24.2
½	cup minced green onion (scallion)	2.4	0.9
1	egg yolk	0.3	3.5
1	teaspoon Worcestershire sauce (optional)	1.0	0
½	teaspoon garlic powder	1.2	0
	salt to taste (about ½ teaspoon)	0	0
	freshly ground black pepper to taste	0	0
⅓	cup Bread Crumbs I (page 25)	3.7	7.6
¼	cup whole almond meal	3.0	6.0
¼	cup unprocessed wheat bran	3.0	2.0
2	tablespoons olive or coconut oil	0	0
	Total	*25.8*	*44.2*

Combine the soybeans and onion in a medium-size mixing bowl. Beat the egg yolk with the Worcestershire sauce, then stir in the garlic powder, salt, and pepper. Stir this mixture into the soybean-onion mixture. Add the bread crumbs, almond meal, and wheat bran, combine thoroughly, and chill the dough for about 15 minutes. Shape the dough into patties so that you get 8 to 10 or however many you want.

Heat a large, heavy skillet on medium. Add coconut or peanut oil. Cook the cakes in the hot oil (reduce heat to low if needed—do not let the patties brown too quickly). Turn each cake once, cooking for about 3 to 4 minutes on each side. Drain the cakes on paper towels and serve.

Variation: Hot Little Soybean Fritters

Follow the recipe for Vegetarian Burgers on page 214, but beat these ingredients: 1 teaspoon dried oregano, ¼ teaspoon ground cinnamon, ¼ teaspoon red pepper flakes, ¼ teaspoon ground cumin, 2 ounces canned chile peppers, diced. This adds 1.0 gram of carb to each serving.

Cauliflower Casserole with Croutons

This casserole turns cauliflower into a lively surprise. Herbed Croutons I (page 24) or gluten-free Herbed Croutons II (page 25) and cheese make all the difference. If you have a batch of croutons made, this casserole is even easier.

PREPARATION TIME: 20 minutes. COOKING AND BAKING TIME: 33 to 43 minutes.

SERVING SIZE: ⅕ total yield. AMOUNT PER SERVING: 5.7 grams of carb, 13.7 grams of protein. NUMBER OF SERVINGS: 5.

		CHO (g)	PRO (g)
16	ounces cauliflower florets	12.8	9.6
6	tablespoons butter (¾ stick)	0	0
	salt to taste (about ½ teaspoon)	0	0
	freshly ground black pepper to taste	0	0
½	teaspoon garlic powder	1.2	0
2	cups Herbed Croutons I (page 24)	7.0	14.2
¾	cup grated Parmesan cheese	3.0	35.7
2	egg yolks	0.6	5.6
⅔	cup light or heavy cream	4.2	3.2
	Total	*28.8*	*68.3*

Preheat oven to 325°F to 350°F; butter or oil a medium-size baking pan or ovenproof casserole dish.

Steam or simmer the cauliflower in a small amount of water until soft yet crunchy (about 8 minutes). Put the hot cauliflower in a mixing bowl. Stir in 4 tablespoons butter, salt, and pepper.

Add the garlic powder, croutons, and all but 3 tablespoons cheese to the cauliflower; stir to combine. Beat the egg yolks and combine with the cream. Add to the cauliflower. Put the mixture in a buttered baking dish. Dot with 2 tablespoons butter and sprinkle with 3 tablespoons cheese. Bake for 25 to 35 minutes or until golden brown on top. Serve immediately.

Variation: Cauliflower Casserole with Ham

Turn this great casserole from a side dish or vegetarian meal into an easy entree. Chop about 12 ounces of lean, baked ham or whatever cooked ham you have on hand into ½-inch pieces and mix into the other ingredients before spooning them into the baking dish. (Avoid honey-cured ham.) This adds about 66.0 grams of protein to the meal. Total protein per serving, based on five, is 26.3 grams. Depending on the ham, there may be a slight increase in carb, perhaps 3.6 grams. Carb count per serving could go up to 6.4 grams.

Variation: **Cauliflower Casserole with Ground Beef**

Here is another way to make an entree out of this dish. When you prepare the casserole, heat a skillet on medium-high and add about 16 ounces lean ground beef to it. Brown the beef, season, and cook until done. Drain thoroughly. Mix with the other casserole ingredients and spoon into the casserole dish. Instead of ground beef, you can use leftover beef roast. Add about 12 ounces of finely chopped roast beef. This adds a total of about 80.0 grams of protein but no carb. A serving, based on five, has 29.1 grams of protein.

Mock Mashed Potatoes

If you miss those heaping helpings of creamy mashed potatoes from long ago with your steak, you're in for a treat with this mock version of the classic. They're so delicious that you'll want to make a big batch, because with carb counts this low you'll want seconds. These mock potatoes go with anything, from a juicy steak to Southern Fried Chicken and Gravy (page 111).

PREPARATION TIME: 15 minutes. COOKING AND BAKING TIME: 40 minutes.
SERVING SIZE: ¼ total yield. AMOUNT PER SERVING: 4.2 grams of carb, 3.2
  grams of protein. NUMBER OF SERVINGS: 4.

		CHO (g)	PRO (g)
20	ounces cauliflower florets	16.0	12.0
2	tablespoons heavy cream	0.8	0.6
2	tablespoons butter, melted (¼ stick)	0	0
1	tablespoon Basic Mayonnaise (page 239)	0	0
½	teaspoon salt (or to taste)	0	0
	white pepper to taste	0	0
1	tablespoon butter	0	0
	Total	*16.8*	*12.6*

Preheat oven to 350°F about 15 minutes before you plan to serve the mock potatoes. Butter or oil a medium baking pan or ovenproof casserole dish.

Steam or simmer the cauliflower for a few minutes or cook in a microwave-safe covered dish with 2 tablespoons of water. Microwave on high for 5 minutes and check. The florets should be very soft. Continue to cook in 1-minute increments until done. Drain cauliflower thoroughly; cool slightly.

Puree the cauliflower in a food processor with all of the remaining ingredients except the 1 tablespoon butter until completely smooth. (In the blender, unless the motor is very powerful, you'll need to puree the cauliflower in batches: Put about half of the cooked florets into the jar of a blender; add half the cream, half the melted butter, half the mayonnaise, half the salt and pepper. Blend on high until smooth.)

Put the puree in the casserole dish and set aside until about 20 minutes before serving time. (If it will be more than an hour, refrigerate.) Dot the top of the mock potatoes with 1 tablespoon butter and bake, uncovered for about 20 minutes. If you're cooking meat, you can reheat the cauliflower alongside it during the last 15 to 20 minutes of cooking time or during the resting period for the meat. Serve hot.

Variation: Crumby Mashed Potatoes

If you want to add some bread crumbs to the cauliflower, stir these ingredients into the puree: 1/3 cup Bread Crumbs I (page 25) or gluten-free Bread Crumbs II (page 26), 1/2 teaspoon garlic powder, 2 tablespoons grated Parmesan cheese. Proceed with the directions. This will increase the servings by one. Based on five servings, each has 4.4 grams of carb and 7.1 grams of protein.

Variation: Mock Shepherd's Pie

This humble meal may become a hot menu item in low-carb households—it is that good. Prepare Mock Mashed Potatoes or the variation (above) and add 2 egg yolks, lightly beaten. Omit the butter. Preheat the oven to 350°F. Prepare 1/2 cup chopped onion. Heat a heavy skillet on medium, then add some olive or coconut oil. Sauté the onion in the hot oil until translucent. Add 1 cup of small button mushrooms without stems to the onion and cook until done, about 5 minutes. Put the onion and mushrooms in a medium-size mixing bowl. Increase heat under the skillet to medium-high; add oil if needed. Quickly brown 16 ounces of lean ground beef and cook until done. Season with salt and freshly ground pepper. Mix the meat with the onion and mushrooms. Butter a glass or other pie pan. Put the meat in the bottom. Sprinkle with 1/4 cup grated Parmesan cheese. Cover with the Mock Mashed Potatoes. Bake for 25 to 30 minutes. Serve with a zesty green salad and Pumpernickel Bread (page 35). This is a main meal for four. One serving has 6.0 grams of carb and 25.0 grams of protein. The protein count is slightly higher if you use the variation.

EGGPLANT GUIDELINES

Eggplants are very useful on a low-carb diet. Not only are they low-carb, like so many veggies, but they have a relatively bland taste and an odd, almost meaty texture. With these qualities, they are sometimes presented in place of pasta or potatoes. Eggplants can add substance and bulk to soups and sauces without introducing a noticeably foreign flavor (it is how they are often used in recipes in this book). Besides, the eggplant can be a nice vegetable in its own right. Some cooks may shy away from eggplants simply because of the bother of having to drain slices or sprinkle them with salt and let them sit. The eggplants most in need of this treatment are big, roundish eggplants that commonly carry loads of seeds. Buy young, shiny, firm, slender specimens. These eggplants rarely need to be drained and are unlikely to be bitter. Eggplants used in this book are usually peeled. You can use them unpeeled if you prefer. Eggplants have 1.0 gram of carb in 1 ounce and 0.3 gram of protein.

Breaded Eggplant Fritters

A coating of Parmesan cheese and bread crumbs makes this eggplant dish delicious and quick to fix. Use Bread Crumbs I (page 25) or gluten-free Bread Crumbs II (page 26).

PREPARATION TIME: 10 minutes. COOKING TIME: 10 minutes.
SERVING SIZE: ½ total yield. AMOUNT PER SERVING: 4.8 grams of carb, 10.3 grams of protein. NUMBER OF SERVINGS: 2.

	CHO (g)	PRO (g)
1 small, firm, peeled eggplant (about 8 ounces)	8.0	5.4
1 egg, beaten	0.6	6.0
⅓ cup Bread Crumbs I or II (page 25 and page 26)	3.7	7.6
1 ounce grated Parmesan cheese (¼ cup)	1.0	11.9
½ cup olive oil or coconut oil for frying	0	0
½ teaspoon garlic powder	1.2	0
salt to taste	0	0
freshly ground black pepper to taste	0	0
2 tablespoons freshly chopped parsley	0	0
Total	*14.5*	*30.9*

Cut the eggplant in ½-inch slices. Set out one bowl with the beaten egg and another with the bread crumbs, cheese, and garlic powder mixed together. Dip each slice of eggplant first in the egg, then in the bread crumbs and cheese mixture. Coat well. Place the coated slices on a platter.

Heat a large, heavy skillet on medium-low. Add the olive or coconut oil. Cook the eggplant in the hot oil until golden brown on both sides, about 4 minutes total. (Do not crowd the slices; you need to be able to turn them.) Low-carb bread crumbs tend to darken faster than standard bread crumbs. Reduce heat, if needed, to keep the slices light golden in color. Sprinkle with salt, pepper, and parsley. Serve immediately.

Eggplant Parmigiana

If you miss eggplant parmigiana—well, now you can eat it again. This is not a quick-to-fix meal, but if you can find the time to do it, you will be rewarded. Serve with Magic Rolls (page 22) or Best Garlic Bread (page 26).

PREPARATION TIME: 45 minutes. BAKING TIME: 30 to 35 minutes.
SERVING SIZE: ⅙ total yield. AMOUNT PER SERVING: 9.5 grams of carb, 26.8 grams of protein. NUMBER OF SERVINGS: 6.

		CHO (g)	PRO (g)
2	medium-size eggplants, peeled (about 18 ounces)	18.0	9.0
4	ounces shredded whole-milk mozzarella cheese	2.8	24.8
5	ounces grated Parmesan cheese	4.0	59.5
4	ounces shredded Swiss cheese (or very thinly sliced)	4.0	32.4
6	tablespoons tomato paste	15.0	6.0
1½	cups dry white wine	2.4	0
½	cup water	0	0
	salt to taste (about ¼ teaspoon)	0	0
	freshly ground black pepper to taste	0	0
2	eggs, beaten	1.2	12.0
¾	cup Bread Crumbs I (page 25)	8.4	17.1
½	teaspoon garlic powder	1.2	0
¼	cup olive oil or coconut oil (more if needed)	0	0
4	tablespoons butter (½ stick), (optional)	0	0
	Total	*57.0*	*160.8*

Butter or oil a 2-quart baking pan or ovenproof casserole dish. Cut the eggplant into ½-inch-thick slices. (Read about eggplant on page 220.) Set out the cheeses and have ready. Mix the tomato paste with the wine and water; stir into a smooth sauce (you can do this in the blender). Season with salt and pepper.

Set out two shallow bowls for the beaten eggs and the bread crumbs. Mix the crumbs with garlic powder and salt. Dip each slice of eggplant first in the eggs, then in the bread crumbs. Coat well. Put the coated slices on a platter.

Heat a large, heavy skillet over medium-low heat. Heat the olive oil. Cook the eggplant slices in the hot oil until golden brown on each side. Do not crowd the slices; you need to be able to turn them. Pre-heat oven to 350°F when you are about halfway through cooking the eggplant. Drain eggplant on paper towels. Transfer the cooked slices to a holding plate until all slices are cooked. Note that these bread crumbs tend to darken faster than standard bread crumbs. Reduce heat if needed to keep the slices light golden in color.

Build the eggplant parmigiana. Put a layer of eggplant (about half) in the bottom of the casserole dish. Sprinkle about half of each of the three cheeses over the eggplant slices, but reserve some Parmesan cheese (to taste) for topping the finished casserole. Pour about half of the sauce over the cheeses. Add the next layer of eggplant slices and repeat the process. Pour the rest of the sauce on top. Sprinkle the casserole with bread crumbs and 1 ounce Parmesan cheese. Dot with butter. Bake the casserole, uncovered, for about 30 to 35 minutes or until light golden brown.

Nutty Green Beans

If you thought there was nothing new you could do with green beans, think again. This smoky, crunchy, peppery, nutty version of the old standard will surprise you with its contrasts of flavors and textures. Good with grilled or roasted meats, this dish sits nicely on the plate beside almost any entree. The recipe can be multiplied easily and reheats well.

PREPARATION TIME: 15 to 20 minutes. COOKING TIME: 12 to 15 minutes. SERVING SIZE: ⅙ total yield. AMOUNT PER SERVING: 3.8 grams of carb, 2.4 grams of protein. NUMBER OF SERVINGS: 6.

	CHO (g)	PRO (g)
1 pound fresh green beans	16.9	8.3
1 tablespoon garlic-flavored olive oil	0	0
½ cup coarsely chopped pecans	2.0	6.0
½ teaspoon finely chopped, dried		
chipotle pepper*	0.2	0
Total	*19.1*	*14.3*

Trim the tough ends from the beans. In a covered saucepan, cook the beans and pepper in about 1 cup of boiling, salted water until tender crisp—about 10 minutes. Drain. In a skillet, heat the olive oil, then add the pecans, and cook them for 45 seconds, stirring constantly to prevent burning as they toast. Add the drained beans. Heat through, stirring constantly to coat with oil, about 1 to 2 minutes. Serve immediately.

* You may substitute ¼ teaspoon cayenne pepper and ¼ teaspoon liquid smoke for the chipotle pepper.

Very Special Mushrooms

If you're a mushroom lover, you're in for a real treat. This easy, cheesy recipe will become one of your staples. The mushrooms pair well with any meat, fish, or poultry entree and can easily be made in larger batches for buffet suppers or when veggies are needed at a potluck dinner.

PREPARATION TIME: 25 to 30 minutes. BAKING TIME: 20 minutes.
SERVING SIZE: ⅙ total yield. AMOUNT PER SERVING: 4.6 grams of carb, 8.1 grams of protein. NUMBER OF SERVINGS: 6.

	CHO (g)	PRO (g)
1 pound white mushrooms	16.0	8.0
1 cup beef broth (page 80)	1.0	3.0
2 teaspoons salt	0	0
2 tablespoons butter (¼ stick)	0	0
½ cup chopped scallion (green and white parts)	2.4	0.9
2 packages frozen spinach (10 ounces each), cooked and drained	3.0	8.0
1 teaspoon black pepper	1.0	0
1 cup grated sharp cheddar cheese	4.0	28.4
Total	*27.4*	*48.3*

Preheat oven to 350°F. Lightly oil or butter an 8- by 11-inch baking dish.

Wipe mushrooms with a damp cloth or paper towel. Cut off the hard stem ends and discard; cut off the rest (and usable) parts of the stems. Chop them coarsely and set aside.

In a medium saucepan, poach the mushroom caps in beef broth plus 1 teaspoon salt until slightly limp.

Heat a skillet on medium-low. Add the butter. When it bubbles (don't brown), add the onion and mushroom stems. Sauté until the onion is transparent, but do not allow it to brown.

Line the bottom of the baking dish with the spinach. Scatter the mushroom stems and onion over this spinach layer, then top with the mushroom caps, cavity-side down. Sprinkle with the remaining salt, pepper, and cheese. Bake until bubbly, about 20 minutes. Serve immediately. .

Braised Mustard Greens

Greens of all types are a low-carber's delight—filled with important nutrients and vitamins and really low on starch and sugars. These greens make a wonderful side dish for Southern Fried Chicken (page 111) with Elegant Biscuits (page 28) and a big glass of iced tea (artificially sweetened, of course).

PREPARATION TIME: 15 to 20 minutes. COOKING TIME: 20 to 30 minutes. SERVING SIZE: ⅙ total yield. AMOUNT PER SERVING: 3.7 grams of carb, 4.5 grams of protein. NUMBER OF SERVINGS: 6.

		CHO (g)	PRO (g)
2	tablespoons olive oil	0	0
6	chopped scallions (green and white parts)	3.6	1.4
2	cloves garlic, minced or pressed	1.8	0
2	tablespoons chicken broth	0.2	0.6
2	pounds mustard greens, rinsed, stemmed, and torn	14.5	24.5
1	tablespoon lime juice (about ½ small lime)	1.3	0
½	teaspoon salt	0	0
	freshly ground black pepper to taste	0	0
	Total	*21.4*	*26.5*

In a large stockpot, heat the oil on medium-low. Add the onion and garlic and cook until golden. Add the chicken broth. Add the mustard greens. Cover and simmer about 20 to 30 minutes or longer, depending on the toughness of the greens. Drain. Put in a serving bowl and add the lime juice, salt, and pepper. Toss to coat evenly before serving.

Grandmother's Turnip Greens

This old-fashioned, Southern side dish pairs perfectly with Southern Fried Chicken (page 111), roast pork, roast beef, grilled sausages, or just about any simply prepared entree. Turnip greens are a must-serve with the traditional black-eyed peas and ham on New Year's Day to ensure luck and good fortune in the coming year. To really serve it the way Grandmother did, once on the plate, you'll want to perk up the greens with a dash or two of "pepper salts" (hot pickled pepper juice). The recipe can be multiplied easily—you're limited only by how large a pot you have to boil the greens in.

PREPARATION TIME: 15 to 20 minutes. COOKING TIME: 1 hour.
SERVING SIZE: ¼ total yield. AMOUNT PER SERVING: 6.0 grams of carb, 4.2 grams of protein. NUMBER OF SERVINGS: 4.

		CHO (g)	PRO (g)
2	pounds fresh turnip greens, trimmed, torn, and washed	23.0	13.6
2	ounces salt pork	0	2.9
1	teaspoon freshly ground black pepper	1.0	0
	salt to taste	0	0
	Total	*23.9*	*16.5*

Wash greens, rinsing several times to remove all grit. With a sharp paring knife, cut away all central stems, as well as any side stem that looks tough. Cut or tear the trimmed leaves into large pieces. Wash again and drain. Soak the salt pork in water for a few minutes to remove some of its saltiness. Rinse and repeat. Cut the rinsed meat into three or four pieces and score each piece.

In a covered saucepan or pot large enough to hold all the greens, bring 2 cups of water to a rolling boil. Add the salt pork pieces and boil for about 10 to 15 minutes.

Add the torn greens and pepper to the pot. Cover, reduce heat to medium, and cook until greens are tender, about 30 to 45 minutes or sometimes longer, depending on the tenderness of the greens you started with. Although the greens are ready to serve, you can continue to simmer for an hour or more if you want. Taste the greens and add salt only if needed—the saltiness of the pork may be sufficient.

Onion Parmesan Gratin

Quick, easy, savory, and a great accompaniment to any meat, fish, poultry, or game dish, this cheesy onion casserole may become a favorite. Made in larger batches, it's great for large get-togethers.

PREPARATION TIME: 20 minutes. COOKING AND BROILING TIME: 13 to 14 minutes.

SERVING SIZE: ⅛ total yield. AMOUNT PER SERVING: 8.7 grams of carb, 5.2 grams of protein. NUMBER OF SERVINGS: 8.

	CHO (g)	PRO (g)
4 tablespoons butter (½ stick)	0	0
2 pounds sweet onions, peeled and thinly sliced	64.0	10.6
¾ teaspoon ground cloves	0.8	0
¼ teaspoon dried thyme	0.5	0
1 teaspoon salt (or to taste)	0	0
2 egg yolks, beaten	0.6	5.6
¼ cup heavy cream	1.6	1.2
½ cup grated Parmesan cheese	2.0	23.8
Total	*69.5*	*41.2*

Preheat broiler or oven on high. Lightly oil an ovenproof gratin or shallow baking dish.

Heat a large, heavy skillet on medium-low. Add butter, but do not let it brown. Add the onion, cloves, thyme, and salt. Cover and cook over low heat until onions are very soft, about 10 minutes. When done, transfer to the oiled gratin or baking dish and spread out evenly.

Meanwhile, in a small bowl, combine the egg yolks with the cream and mix well. Stir in the cheese and pour the mixture over the onions. Broil about 2 inches from the heat until the top sizzles and browns, about 3 minutes. Serve immediately.

Pepper Pots

These colorful baked stuffed peppers will work especially well with fish or chicken entrees that tend to be more delicate in flavor and in need of a pick-me-up. You'll love them for buffet suppers or as a side dish for meats.

PREPARATION TIME: 25 to 30 minutes. BAKING TIME: 35 minutes.
SERVING SIZE: ½ stuffed pepper. AMOUNT PER SERVING: 6.8 grams of carb, 3.5 grams of protein. NUMBER OF SERVINGS: 12.

		CHO (g)	PRO (g)
24	anchovy fillets	0	27.8
6	large green bell peppers	30.0	6.0
12	cloves garlic, minced or pressed	10.8	2.4
24	cherry tomatoes, quartered	14.4	3.5
2	medium yellow bell peppers, cored, seeded, and chopped	10.5	2.1
2	tablespoons freshly chopped thyme	0.5	0
¼	cup olive oil	0	0
2	teaspoons salt (or as desired)	0	0
2	teaspoons freshly ground black pepper	2.0	0.6
¾	cup balsamic vinegar	13.9	0
	Total	*82.1*	*42.4*

Preheat oven to 425°F. Butter or oil a medium-size baking pan or ovenproof casserole dish.

Remove the anchovy fillets from the jar or can and soak them in about ¼ cup milk in a small bowl for 20 to 30 minutes prior to use. Rinse them thoroughly in cold water. This process removes the intensely salty, fishy taste from them. If you like this taste, you may omit this step.

Cut the green bell peppers in half lengthwise to create the "pots." Remove pith and seeds, taking care that you do not puncture the pots or they will leak. Try to leave the stem in place, again to prevent leaking.

Arrange the pepper pots cut-side up, and brush the interior and top of each pot with a little olive oil. In the bottom of each pot, place two well-rinsed anchovy fillets, forming a circle. Place one minced clove of garlic in the center of each anchovy circle.

In a medium-size bowl, mix the tomatoes and yellow peppers and divide this mixture evenly between the 12 pots. Sprinkle the top of each pot with the fresh thyme and drizzle each pot with about ½ teaspoon olive oil. Season each pot with salt and pepper. Bake the pepper pots for 35 minutes. Remove from oven and let stand to cool slightly and settle. Drizzle each pot with about 1½ teaspoons balsamic vinegar before serving.

Yellow Crookneck Squash Casserole

This easy, tasty recipe for squash will become a favorite. It works well for buffet suppers or simply for the family. It can be made just prior to serving, but this dish also reheats well. It can become a side dish on consecutive evenings or appear for lunch the next day. It's so low in carbs, you could have two servings and still have carb room to spare!

PREPARATION TIME: 20 minutes. BAKING TIME: 20 minutes.
SERVING SIZE: 1/10 total yield. AMOUNT PER SERVING: 1.7 grams of carb, 3.3 grams of protein. NUMBER OF SERVINGS: 10.

	CHO (g)	PRO (g)
5 cups sliced yellow crookneck squash	9.5	3.0
8 tablespoons butter (1 stick)	0	0
¾ cup chopped scallions, white part only	3.6	1.4
2 eggs, beaten	1.2	12.0
¾ cup plain pork rinds, crushed (about 12 rinds)	0	7.3
1 teaspoon salt (or to taste)	0	0
½ teaspoon black pepper	0.5	0
½ teaspoon garlic powder	1.2	0
½ teaspoon dried thyme	0.3	0
3 tablespoons grated Parmesan cheese	0.8	8.9
Total	*17.1*	*32.6*

Preheat oven to 350°F; butter or oil a medium-size baking pan or ovenproof casserole dish.

In a fairly large covered saucepan, cook the squash in about 1 cup of boiling salted water until tender, about 12 minutes. Drain well and mash the squash with a potato masher or fork. Set aside.

Heat a small skillet on medium-high heat; add the butter. When the butter foams and before it browns, add the onions and sauté until limp.

Add the onion, eggs, pork rinds, and seasonings to the mashed squash. Mix well. Spoon squash mixture into the casserole dish. Bake, uncovered, for about 20 minutes. Remove from oven and sprinkle cheese on top. Return to oven and bake until the cheese melts and browns slightly.

Variation: Crumby Crookneck Casserole

Although Bread Crumbs I (page 25) or gluten-free Bread Crumbs II (page 26) cannot replace the special flavor of the pork rinds, you can use about ⅓ cup crumbs in place of the rinds if you like. You come closer in taste to the pork rinds by increasing grated Parmesan cheese to 4 tablespoons and garlic powder to 1 teaspoon. All of this adds less than 1.0 gram of carb per serving. You can virtually ignore it.

Variation: Mock Sweet Potato Casserole

For most of you, the high-carb version of this dish has been painfully absent from many meals, especially Thanksgiving; this delicious low-carb mockery of the real thing will delight you. You still need to be careful, though. Preheat oven to 350°F. Follow the directions for boiling 5 cups sliced yellow crookneck squash, but salt sparingly or not at all. Drain. Butter a medium-size baking pan or casserole dish and put the squash in it. Melt 1 stick of butter (4 ounces) in microwave. Add the following: 2 tablespoons lemon juice (2.6 grams of carb), 2 tablespoons brown sugar (24.0 grams of carb), and 5 packets Splenda sugar substitute (or to taste). The syrup and the squash combined have 45.2 grams of carb. The amount of protein is negligible. One serving has 4.5 grams of carb. You can leave out the brown sugar and use about 12 or more packets of Splenda. That drops the count per serving to a much more reasonable 2.9 grams of carb. Pour one-half of the syrup over the squash and bake for about 10 minutes. Add the other half of the syrup after 15 minutes. Bake the dish for a total of about 35 minutes.

Zucchini Fritters

These crispy little patties work well with everything from steak, fish, and chicken to breakfast eggs and omelets. Anywhere you'd serve a side of hash brown potatoes, you can substitute Zucchini Fritters. They're so good, we'd opt for them over potatoes even if the carb counts weren't so low.

PREPARATION TIME: 15 to 20 minutes. COOKING TIME: 6 to 10 minutes.
SERVING SIZE: ¼ total yield. AMOUNT PER SERVING: 2.9 grams of carb,
   5.9 grams of protein. NUMBER OF SERVINGS: 4.

	CHO (g)	PRO (g)
3 medium zucchini, skin on, grated	10.0	6.8
2 eggs, beaten	1.2	12.0
½ cup plain pork rinds, crushed		
(about 8 rinds)	0	4.9
1 teaspoon salt	0	0
½ teaspoon black pepper	0.5	0
3 tablespoons coconut oil	0	0
Total	*11.7*	*23.7*

Place the grated zucchini in a colander and sprinkle with salt. Allow it to sit at room temperature for 10 minutes to draw out excess water. Pat dry with lots of paper towels.

In a medium-size mixing bowl, combine the eggs, pork rinds, salt, and pepper. Add the grated squash and mix thoroughly.

Melt the coconut oil in a heavy skillet. Drop the zucchini mixture by heaping tablespoonfuls into the hot oil and flatten with a spatula. Work in batches if necessary so you don't crowd the pan. Fry for a few minutes (until they begin to brown on the bottom), then turn, frying until brown on both sides. Drain on paper towels and serve.

Variation: Crumby Fritters

Crushed pork rinds give a savory, smoky flavor to fritters. Although you cannot achieve the same flavor, you can substitute ½ cup Bread Crumbs I (page 25). This will raise carb grams per serving by 1.4 grams and protein to 7.5 grams.

8

LOW-CARB COMFORT FOOD SAUCES AND SALAD DRESSINGS

A good sauce can make a meal—what's Southern fried chicken and biscuits without the gravy? But, because many gravies and sauces call for thickening with flour, corn starch, or a roux, the carb counts make them a dangerous temptation to the low-carb devotee. In this chapter, you'll learn methods for thickening sauces and gravies with an unusual variety of foods, including eggplant, egg, low-carb bread crumbs, and even black soybeans.

We've included several recipes for salad dressings. Here you may well ask yourself why, with the hundreds of commercial dressings that line the shelves of every market, would you need to make your own? The answer is simple: if you make it yourself, you have control not only over the carb content by avoiding sugars and starchy thickeners but over the quality of oil. Most commercial dressings—from salad dressings to mayonnaise—contain soybean oil, a major source of unlabeled *trans* fats, known to damage health. Even in the case of potentially good oils, such as canola oil, the deodorizing process can damage the oil so that up to 40 or even 50 percent of the ALA (a type of fatty acid richly present in canola oil) can be converted into the *trans* configuration, turning what might have been good into a bottle or jar of something of less quality (to put it mildly). So don't sacrifice your good health for convenience. Once you get the hang of it, it takes very little time to make your own salad dressings, cocktail sauces, mayonnaise, and gravy. And with the flavor and quality you get in return, we think it simply doesn't make sense not to make your own.

Basic Vinaigrette

Combine oil with lemon juice or vinegar—and there is vinaigrette. This combination of acid and oil is all some folks dribble on a salad. If you use high-quality vinegar and oil, the result can be very tasty. Most folks like to add other flavors to a vinaigrette and mix it all up. It takes only minutes to make this, so there is no need to go for volume. Keep all dressings in the fridge and remove shortly before using. (If you forget, run hot water over the bottle for a few seconds if the dressing is too thick to pour.) You can decide whether you want it thin, with the oil on top, requiring you to shake the dressing, or you can create a suspension or emulsion. To emulsify, beat all ingredients except the oil with a wire whisk for a few seconds before adding the oil. Dribble the oil into the mixture while beating, and a creamy dressing will ensue.

PREPARATION TIME: 5 minutes.

SERVING SIZE: ⅓ total yield. AMOUNT PER SERVING: 1.1 grams of carb, no protein. NUMBER OF SERVINGS: 3.

	CHO (g)	PRO (g)
2 tablespoons white wine vinegar	0	0
1 tablespoon balsamic vinegar*	2.0	0
1 clove garlic, minced (or ¼ teaspoon garlic powder)	0.9	0
½ teaspoon Dijon-type mustard	0.5	0
4 tablespoons extra-virgin olive oil (or oil of choice)	0	0
salt to taste (about ¼ teaspoon)	0	0
freshly ground black pepper	0	0
Total	*3.4*	*0*

Put all of the ingredients except oil in a small bowl and stir or beat for a few seconds with a wire whisk. Add oil. Put the dressing in a bottle and shake before using. For a creamy vinaigrette, beat the basic ingredients except oil for about 10 seconds, then add the oil very slowly, beating constantly.

Variation: Herb Vinaigrette

Follow the recipe for Basic Vinaigrette above, but add ¼ teaspoon freshly ground sage and ¼ teaspoon freshly ground marjoram or

---

* Balsamic vinegar tastes good but does have carbs. You can substitute a good wine vinegar and save the 2.0 grams, if you like.

small amounts of any fresh or dried herb. The change in carb grams is insignificant. You can vary the herbs on your own. Experiment with different herb flavors, if you like.

Variation: Caper Vinaigrette

Follow the recipe for Basic Vinaigrette on page 236, but omit the mustard. Add 1 teaspoon freshly chopped chives and 1 tablespoon crushed capers. The change in carbs is insignificant.

Variation: Sesame Dressing

This dressing is especially delicious if you serve it with seafood. Look for dark sesame oil (it's made from roasted sesame seeds). It has a strong but delicious flavor. You probably won't be using this dressing often; make it in a small quantity. Follow the recipe for Basic Vinaigrette on page 236, but increase the lemon juice to 2 tablespoons and delete mustard. Use 2 tablespoons dark sesame oil and 3 tablespoons light olive oil in place of the extra-virgin olive oil. Sprinkle 2 tablespoons roasted sesame seeds over the salad after you have added the dressing. Mix well. If you roast your own sesame seeds, heat a small skillet on medium. Add the sesame seeds and stir constantly. Some will pop up as they toast. Stir them for about 1 minute. Do not let them get dark.

Variation: Peanut Dressing

Follow the recipe for Basic Vinaigrette on page 236, but mix 2 tablespoons peanut oil with 2 tablespoons light olive oil in place of the extra-virgin olive oil. Add 1 teaspoon soy sauce. Roast 1 tablespoon raw peanuts in a dry skillet over medium heat for a few minutes, until brown. Keep stirring. Cool nuts and chop or crush. Use a mezzaluna or put the nuts in a small plastic bag and crush with a mallet. Sprinkle the nuts over the salad before you add the dressing.

Hail of a Caesar Dressing

Nothing tastes quite as good with savory meats, poultry, or fish as the tang of a good Caesar salad. Whereas making the dressing the traditional way—with raw egg—might seem daunting, this quick and easy version takes no time to prepare and tastes so much like the real McCoy that you'll find yourself looking around for the skilled waiter with the tableside preparation cart. Our thanks—and yours, once you've tried it—go to Michael Judd, a friend and fellow physician from Spokane, Washington, who developed this recipe that will make your friends envious of your culinary expertise. The recipe can be multiplied easily and will keep in the refrigerator, tightly sealed, for a couple of days.

SERVING SIZE: ¼ total yield. AMOUNT PER SERVING: 2.0 grams of carb, 0.7 gram of protein. NUMBER OF SERVINGS: 4.

		CHO (g)	PRO (g)
1	lemon, juice only	2.4	0
1	clove garlic, minced or pressed	0.9	0
4	anchovy fillets, mashed	0	1.4
1	tablespoon Basic Mayonnaise (page 239)	0	0
1	tablespoon Dijon-style mustard	1.5	1.5
1	tablespoon Worcestershire sauce	3.0	0
	Total	7.8	2.9

Put the juice of 1 lemon into a shallow bowl. Add the garlic. Add the anchovy fillets and mash with two forks until you've got a smooth paste (or use anchovy paste equal to 4 anchovies—about 1 to 1½ teaspoons—and stir to blend).

Add the remaining ingredients and mix with a fork to blend thoroughly. When you serve dressed greens, you can put a couple of whole anchovy fillets and/or Herbed Croutons I or II (page 24 and page 25) on top, if desired.

Basic Mayonnaise

It is easy to make a terrific mayonnaise in 5 minutes or less. So it is really more a matter of getting in the habit of doing it. Use a fairly neutral oil for the basic mayonnaise, such as a good-quality, pure, light olive oil. Mayonnaise is always made with egg. The egg helps create the emulsion and turns the dressing into this astonishing, creamy wonder that it is. Salmonella contamination of eggs is a relatively rare occurrence, but it does happen. If this concerns you, you can simply substitute pasteurized eggs for the egg yolks. You need a food processor or blender to make mayonnaise.

PREPARATION TIME: 3 to 5 minutes.
SERVING SIZE: 1 tablespoon. AMOUNT PER SERVING: negligible amount of carb and protein. NUMBER OF SERVINGS: 24.

	CHO (g)	PRO (g)
2 egg yolks*	0.6	5.6
1 teaspoon Dijon-style mustard	0.5	0
2 teaspoons lemon juice	0.9	0
1 tablespoon white wine vinegar	0	0
½ teaspoon salt (or to taste)	0	0
freshly ground white pepper to taste	0	0
trace of cayenne pepper	0	0
1 cup light olive oil	0	0
Total	2.0	5.6

Put the egg yolks, mustard, lemon juice, vinegar, salt, pepper, and cayenne in the bowl of a food processor or blender. Briefly blend the ingredients, but they should be well blended. Add the oil gradually, in a very thin stream, with the processor (or blender) running. When all the oil has been incorporated, check the mayonnaise. If it is too stiff, close the lid, turn the appliance back on, and add about a tablespoon of hot water. Always refrigerate mayonnaise.

Variation: Low-Carb Tartar Sauce

Follow the directions for making Basic Mayonnaise (above). To every ½ cup of Basic Mayonnaise add 2 teaspoons chopped drained capers, 1 teaspoon fresh minced chives, 1 teaspoon lemon juice, and 1 tablespoon finely chopped dill pickles. Combine and stir. The total addition of carbs is only about 1.7 grams.

Variation: Low-Carb Green Goddess Dressing

Follow the directions for making Basic Mayonnaise (page 239). For every ½ cup of Green Goddess Dressing you want, add 1 minced anchovy fillet (or ½ teaspoon anchovy paste), ¼ teaspoon garlic powder, 1 tablespoon finely chopped green onion, 1 tablespoon freshly chopped parsley, 3 tablespoons sour cream, and salt and freshly ground pepper to taste. Combine and stir.

Variation: Mayonnaise for Fruit Salad

Follow the directions for making Basic Mayonnaise (page 239). Beat ½ cup whipping cream (3.2 grams of carb, 2.4 grams of protein) and mix with ⅔ cup Basic Mayonnaise. Use within 1 hour. This makes about 1⅓ cups. That's about 0.1 grams of carb per tablespoon.

Variation: Curried Mayonnaise

Follow directions for Basic Mayonnaise (page 239). Add 1 tablespoon curry powder (or to taste) and a pinch of ground cumin and cayenne pepper to each 1 cup of mayonnaise. Combine and stir.

Note: To use pasteurized eggs instead of the fresh yolks, replace them with ¼ cup of pasteurized egg white or whole egg substitute. Unless you use egg substitute elsewhere in your cooking, buy the smallest amount of pasteurized eggs available (egg whites often come in ½-cup cartons). Once a carton has been opened, its content must be used within 7 days of that date.

Blue Cheese Dressing

A rich, popular dressing that you can use on many occasions. The better the quality of the blue cheese, the better the dressing.

PREPARATION TIME: 10 minutes.

SERVING SIZE: 2 tablespoons. AMOUNT PER SERVING: 1.1 grams of carb, 2.4 grams of protein. NUMBER OF SERVINGS: 12.

	CHO (g)	PRO (g)
½ cup Basic Mayonnaise (page 239)	0	0
1 teaspoon Dijon-style mustard	0.5	0.5
4 ounces blue cheese	4.0	24.0
½ cup sour cream	4.0	3.2
½ teaspoon salt	0	0
2 tablespoons lemon juice	2.6	0
1 teaspoon Worcestershire sauce	1.0	0
freshly ground white pepper to taste	0	0
salt to taste	0	0
¼ cup light cream	1.6	1.2
Total	*13.7*	*28.9*

Stir all of the ingredients together in a jar and mix well. You can use a blender or food processor, but pulse only once or briefly to maintain the coarse texture of the crumbled blue cheese. The dressing improves in flavor as it ripens.

Honey Mustard Dressing

Regular honey mustard dressing comes with a big carbohydrate price tag (about 20 grams in 2 tablespoons). This one gives you a honey taste for just 2.6 grams of carb in 2 tablespoons.

PREPARATION TIME: 5 minutes.

SERVING SIZE: 2 tablespoons. AMOUNT PER SERVING: 2.6 grams of carb, no protein. NUMBER OF SERVINGS: 8.

	CHO (g)	PRO (g)
1 tablespoon honey	17.0	0
3 tablespoons hot water	0	0
1 tablespoon white wine vinegar	0	0
½ cup Basic Mayonnaise (page 239)	0	0
¼ cup light cream	1.6	1.2
1 packet Splenda sugar substitute (or to taste)	1.0	0
2 teaspoons Dijon-style mustard	1.0	1.0
salt to taste	0	0
freshly ground pepper (white or black) to taste	0	0
Total	*20.6*	*2.2*

Dissolve the honey in the hot water. Stir well. Put all of the other ingredients in a small mixing bowl. Add the dissolved honey. Whisk lightly until smooth. Refrigerate. This dressing keeps for about a week.

Tom's Low-Carb Ketchup

One tablespoon of most ketchups have 4.0 grams of carb. Some dietary ketchups have 2.0 grams per tablespoon, but they're made with aspartame.* This ketchup recipe is great and has only 0.7 gram of carb per tablespoon. You can enjoy ketchup again, even on a low-carb diet.

PREPARATION TIME: 10 minutes.
SERVING SIZE: 1 tablespoon. AMOUNT PER SERVING: 0.7 gram of carb, negligible amount of protein. NUMBER OF SERVINGS: 33.

		CHO (gm)	PRO (gm)
½	cup cubed eggplant	2.0	0
14.5	ounces diced tomatoes, drained†	10.5	3.5
3	tablespoons tomato paste	7.5	3.0
¼	cup red wine vinegar	0	0
2	teaspoons olive oil	0	0
½	teaspoon dried, minced onion	0.9	0
3	packets Splenda sugar substitute	3.0	0
	salt to taste (about ¼ teaspoon or more)	0	0
	Total:	*23.9*	*6.5*

Steam or simmer eggplant in small amount of water until soft, about 6 to 8 minutes. Let cool. Put eggplant and all other ingredients in a food processor or blender and blend until smooth. Adjust seasoning. You can add small amounts of vinegar if you like a sharper taste. Store in fridge. This ketchup will keep for a week or so. You can also freeze it.

* We no longer recommend the use of aspartame. Studies have shown it may be harmful to the brain.

† The taste of this ketchup will be affected by the tomatoes and tomato paste you choose. It's worthwhile to experiment with brands. The carb counts here are based on diced tomatoes that have 3.0 grams of carb per ½ cup serving and tomato paste that has 5.0 grams of carb in 2 tablespoons.

Low-Carb Cocktail Sauce

Cocktail sauce, delicious with seafood, requires tons of ketchup, which is a no-no on a low-carb diet. This one, however, made with low-carb ketchup, is guilt-free and delicious.

PREPARATION TIME: 15 minutes.

SERVING SIZE: 1 tablespoon. AMOUNT PER SERVING: 0.8 gram of carb, negligible amount of protein. NUMBER OF SERVINGS: 16.

	CHO (g)	PRO (g)
⅔ cup Tom's Low-Carb Ketchup (page 243)	7.5	3.3
3 tablespoons lemon juice	3.9	0
1 teaspoon Dijon-style mustard	0.5	0.5
1 tablespoon creamed horseradish	0	0
salt to taste	0	0
freshly ground black pepper to taste	0	0
2 drops Tabasco sauce	0	0
1 teaspoon Worcestershire sauce	1.0	0
Total	*12.9*	*3.8*

Put all of the ingredients in a blender or food processor and blend or process—or simply whisk the sauce together in a small bowl with a wire whisk. This sauce keeps in the fridge for about 10 days—or you may freeze it.

Horseradish Sauce

This is the speediest sauce you can make. Most recipes ask you to whip cream and mix it with horseradish when that standing rib roast is beckoning. Instead, just mix the horseradish with sour cream. It is thick, delicious, and the perfect consistency without extra fuss. (If you want to thin the sauce a bit, just stir in a small amount of heavy cream. Mix just the right amount you need for a meal—you can do it virtually at serving time.

PREPARATION TIME: 2 minutes.

SERVING SIZE: 2 tablespoons. AMOUNT PER SERVING: 1.0 gram of carb, 0.8 gram of protein. NUMBER OF SERVINGS: 4.

	CHO (g)	PRO (g)
½ cup sour cream	4.0	3.2
2 teaspoons prepared horseradish (or to taste)	0	0
salt to taste	0	0
freshly ground black pepper to taste	0	0
Total	*4.0*	*3.2*

Stir together the sour cream and horseradish. Season with salt and pepper. Refrigerate until ready to use.

Cucumber Dill Sauce

Refreshing, zesty, great over meat or fish and also as a dressing—and it's a 5-minute job. Plan on making it ahead, though; it needs to ripen in the fridge for a couple of hours.

PREPARATION TIME: 5 minutes.

SERVING SIZE: ⅕ total yield. AMOUNT PER SERVING: 1.2 grams of carb, negligible amount of protein. NUMBER OF SERVINGS: 5.

	CHO (g)	PRO (g)
½ cup finely chopped cucumber (peeled and seeded)	1.0	0
⅓ cup Basic Mayonnaise (page 239)	0	0
½ cup sour cream	4.0	0
3 teaspoons freshly chopped dill	1.5	0.6
salt to taste	0	0
freshly ground black pepper to taste	0	0
Total	*6.5*	*0.6*

Keep the cucumbers on paper towels in the refrigerator for about 15 minutes or until close to serving time. Mix all of the other ingredients together in a small bowl and refrigerate them for a couple of hours. Add the cucumber to the mixture and stir. Adjust seasonings and serve.

Barbecue Sauce

This is a delicious barbecue sauce you can whip up quickly and use to baste spareribs as they bake.

PREPARATION TIME: 10 minutes. COOKING TIME: 45 minutes.
SERVING SIZE: ⅙ total yield. AMOUNT PER SERVING: 4.6 grams of carb, negligible amount of protein. NUMBER OF SERVINGS: 6.

	CHO (g)	PRO (g)
1 cup canned diced tomatoes	6.0	2.0
½ cup finely chopped onion	5.5	0.9
2 cloves garlic, minced		
(or ½ teaspoon garlic powder)	1.8	0
¼ cup white wine vinegar	0	0
2 teaspoons hickory smoke liquid	6.0	0
4 packets Splenda sugar substitute		
(or to taste)	4.0	0
2 teaspoons chili powder	1.0	0.6
1 teaspoon mustard	0	0
1 tablespoon Worcestershire sauce	3.0	0
salt to taste	0	0
freshly ground black pepper to taste	0	0
Total	*27.3*	*3.5*

Combine all of the ingredients in a 2-quart saucepan and simmer on very low for about 45 minutes. Stir often. You can prepare this sauce up to several days ahead of time. Chill until needed or freeze.

Jiffy Hollandaise Sauce

It's one of those delicious sauces that's usually hard to make and that used to be off limits, anyway. Now you can enjoy the buttery sauce within reason, and this version is a quickie. Serve it over steamed asparagus or anything you like—it always tastes great. Instead of steaming yourself over a water bath (double boiler), whip up this sauce right away when you are ready to serve.

PREPARATION TIME: 5 minutes.

SERVING SIZE: 3 tablespoons. AMOUNT PER SERVING: 0.6 gram of carb, 2.1 grams of protein. NUMBER OF SERVINGS: 4.

		CHO (g)	PRO (g)
3	egg yolks	0.9	8.4
	salt to taste (about ¼ teaspoon)	0	0
	freshly ground black pepper to taste	0	0
	trace of ground cumin (optional)	0	0
1	tablespoon lemon juice	1.3	0
1	tablespoon water	0	0
4	ounces butter (1 stick), melted	0	0
	Total	2.2	8.4

Put the egg yolks in a blender. Add the salt, pepper, and cumin (if used). Do not turn on blender yet.

Add the lemon juice and water to the melted butter. Turn on the blender, mixing the eggs for 30 seconds, then dribble the butter mixture into the blender slowly in a very thin stream. Adjust seasonings and serve immediately. You may also keep it hot in a double boiler over hot (never boiling) water until you need to serve it.

Quickie Mustard Sauce

You will be surprised by what this sauce will do for just about any kind of fish, but it is not limited to fish! This is a sturdy, no-fail, quick sauce—just right for the cook on the run.

PREPARATION TIME: 5 minutes.
SERVING SIZE: ½ cup. AMOUNT PER SERVING: 3.3 grams of carb, 1.5 grams of protein. NUMBER OF SERVINGS: 2.

		CHO (g)	PRO (g)
4	tablespoons butter (½ stick)	0	0
3	teaspoons Dijon-style mustard or to taste	1.5	1.5
2	tablespoons lemon juice	2.6	0
½	cup stock (see page 80)	0.5	1.5
1	teaspoon Wondra flour	1.9	0
	salt to taste	0	0
	freshly ground black pepper to taste	0	0
2	teaspoons freshly chopped parsley	0	0
	Total	*6.5*	*3.0*

Put the butter, mustard, lemon juice, and stock in a small saucepan. Heat on medium. Before the sauce comes to a simmer, sprinkle the Wondra flour over it and whisk it in quickly. Simmer on very low for about 2 minutes. Season with salt and pepper to taste. Keep hot until ready to serve, mixing in parsley just before serving, or keep refrigerated until you need it; you can reheat it in the microwave if you like. If you want the sauce to be a bit thicker, allow it to simmer and reduce until it is right.

Variation: Quickie Mushroom Sauce

Follow the directions for Quickie Mustard Sauce above, but omit the lemon juice and mustard. Increase stock to ¾ cup instead of ½ cup. Reserve 1 tablespoon of butter. Prepare the sauce and set aside. Heat a small skillet on medium, add the reserved tablespoon of butter, then add ¼ cup chopped onion to the hot (but not browned) butter. Sauté for a minute and add ½ cup small button mushrooms without the tough stem parts. Cook until the mushrooms are tender, about 4 minutes. Add onion and mushrooms to the sauce and heat. You can add ¼ cup heavy cream to this sauce if you like. Adjust seasonings. The carb count per serving is 2.1 grams of carb and negligible protein.

Variation: Quickie Lemon Sauce

Follow the directions for Quickie Mustard Sauce on page 249, but omit the mustard. Stir in ⅓ cup light or heavy cream at the end and heat through. This sauce is wonderful with chicken and shrimp. It has about the same carb count as the mustard sauce.

Variation: Quickie Curry Sauce

Follow the directions for Quickie Mustard Sauce on page 249, but omit the mustard and use only 2 teaspoons lemon juice and add ½ cup light or heavy cream and 1 tablespoon curry powder (or to taste). Here's the order: Combine the butter, flour, and curry powder in the saucepan. Stir until the butter has melted and the mixture is smooth. Slowly add the lemon juice, stock, salt, and pepper. Add parsley at the end. This sauce has the same carb count as the Quickie Mustard Sauce. If you want an easy meal that tastes great and a little different, put some salad or popcorn shrimp in the sauce and heat through. Use about 8 to 10 ounces of shrimp and make sure the shrimp, fresh or frozen, smell absolutely fresh. Soak them in ½ cup milk for 10 minutes. Blot them absolutely dry or the sauce will become watery. Adjust seasonings. The carb count is about the same as for the Quickie Mustard Sauce.

Who Doesn't Like Gravy?

There you are with that big turkey. Once upon a time, you may have made a rich, thick gravy to go along with it, for some the best part of the meal. Not to mention the potatoes and stuffing that you could pour the gravy on. This recipe helps you restore those old days. You can have gravy with mashed potatoes (see Mock Mashed Potatoes on page 218), and not just one but several wonderful stuffings (see Chapter 5). Make Cranberry Sauce (page 299) and finish with Best Pumpkin Pie (page 288).

PREPARATION TIME: 20 minutes. COOKING TIME: 10 minutes.
SERVING SIZE: ½ cup. AMOUNT PER SERVING: 3.4 grams of carb, 5.1 grams of protein. NUMBER OF SERVINGS: 6 to 7.

	CHO (g)	PRO (g)
3½ ounces turkey giblets	2.0	19.0
2 cups stock from giblets	2.0	6.0
6 tablespoons butter (¾ stick), (or as desired)	0	0
4 teaspoons Wondra flour	7.7	0
½ cup pan juice from turkey	0.5	1.5
5 ounces peeled and cubed eggplant	5.0	1.5
½ cup heavy cream	3.2	2.4
salt to taste	0	0
freshly ground black pepper to taste	0	0
Total	*20.4*	*30.4*

Clean the giblets and simmer, covered, in about 2 cups of salted water for 1 hour or longer. Drain. Reserve broth. Chop giblets and save in fridge.

Heat a heavy-bottomed saucepan on medium-low, then add the butter. When it foams, add the Wondra flour and stir until it browns slightly. Gradually add about half of the giblet stock and stir until the sauce thickens.

Add the remaining broth along with ½ cup of clear juice from the pan in which you roasted the bird (avoid turkey fat unless the turkey is organic). Add the eggplant to the gravy and simmer for about 10 or 12 minutes until the eggplant is tender.

Put the eggplant chunks along with some gravy in a food processor or blender. Process until smooth. Return to the saucepan. Stir in the cream. Season with salt and pepper. For added flavor, it sometimes helps to add 1 teaspoon of Better Than Bouillon to the gravy. This adds 1.0 gram of carb. Add the chopped giblets and heat through. Serve immediately.

Variation: Jiffy Gravy for Two

There are lots of occasions when just a touch of gravy would hit the spot. Have a roast chicken in the oven? You don't need any gravy— but it is still nice to have and goes well with Mock Mashed Potatoes (page 218) or over Magic Rolls (page 22) or anything else. Pour juice from the chicken (with all fat removed unless organically grown) in a small saucepan and combine with enough water to make 1 cup. Add ½ teaspoon Better Than Bouillon concentrate. Add 2 tablespoons butter. Heat over medium heat. Before the liquid simmers, sprinkle 2 teaspoons Wondra flour over the top and whisk until smooth. Add salt and freshly ground black pepper to taste. Simmer for about 2 minutes; this will reduce the gravy slightly. Serve. This serves 3 to 4, and the total carb count per serving is 2.5 grams. If you just want to make a generic gravy, simply add 1 teaspoon of Better Than Bouillon to 1 cup of water and follow the directions as given. Carbs remain about the same.

THE EGGPLANT AS THICKENER

The eggplant has a bland flavor and a meaty texture. These attributes, not loved by everybody, make it a good substitute for flour in thickening sauces, soups, and other dishes. As a rule of thumb, use 1 cup of peeled, cubed eggplant to thicken 1 cup of liquid. Cook the eggplant until soft, about 10 to 12 minutes. If you want the sauce or soup you are thickening to be smooth, puree the cooked eggplant with a little of the liquid in which it was cooked in a processor or blender until smooth. Otherwise (as in Mock Marinara Sauce on page 134, just cut the eggplant in about ½-inch cubes and allow it to cook with the other ingredients. One cup of peeled, cubed eggplant has 3.0 grams of carb and 0.8 grams of protein; it thickens 1 cup of liquid.

Variation: Black Soybeans as Thickener

Follow the directions in "The Eggplant as Thickener," but substitute ⅓ cup finely mashed black soybeans for the eggplant. The black soybeans add 2.1 grams of carb to 1 cup of liquid and a negligible amount of protein.

9

LOW-CARB
COMFORT FOOD
DESSERTS

In the past, committing to a low-carb lifestyle meant saying a whole host of good-byes: bye-bye to chocolate chip cookies, soft and warm from the oven; so long to frosted sugar or spice cookies at the holidays; adios to cheesecake or pumpkin pie. No thanks to pound cake or peach cobblers. Oh sure, you could splurge on a big celebration and treat yourself to a tiny square of cake . . . or throw caution to the wind and go face first into a really big piece and pay the price of your carb excess the next morning. But if you made a habit of such indulgences, you knew you would find your waistline expanding and your cholesterol, blood sugar, and/or blood pressure on the rise again in no time.

Those days are now gone. Armed with the easy-to-prepare recipes in this chapter and a good cookie sheet, the aroma of baking chocolate chip cookies will again fill your kitchen. And you can be guilt-free, because these cookies have the taste of the original minus the heavy carb load. A coconut cake with frosting for your birthday? No problem—just get the candles ready.

And how long has it been since you enjoyed a thick slice of warm apple pie à la mode without feeling a twinge of guilt? If you've struggled with your weight or with weight-related health issues, it's probably been longer than you care to remember. But now you can enjoy such pleasures again. You'll be making pies with crusts so flaky that you'll swear they can't be low-carb—but they are! And with carb counts this low, guilty feelings won't even enter your mind.

You'll want to remember, of course, that low in carb doesn't mean low in calories, and if you're still in the weight-loss phase of your low-carb regimen, you'll want to eat reasonable portions of these items until you're ready to maintain. If you try to eat an entire key lime pie each evening, for instance, you'll probably stall your weight loss. (In fact, we'll guarantee it.) But once you've reached your weight or health goals, you can enjoy bigger portions more often.

Just knowing you can have a legal pleasure, whether it's a serving of Apple Brown Betty or a bowl of low-carb Ice Cream, can make the difference between success and failure in staying with any nutritional regimen. These recipes are designed to make it really easy for you to live low-carb for the long haul by filling that big empty tray on the dessert cart. Enjoy!

Best Almond Biscotti

Biscotti are baked twice. The end result is a hard, dry cookie that tastes great with coffee. It sounds like double the work but really isn't. You bake miniloaves and slice them, then you bake the slices as if they were cookies, which they become. Biscotti last virtually indefinitely, even at room temperature. If you want, you can add a touch of a Sugar Glaze (page 275) or a Chocolate-Flavored Glaze (page 275). This adds 0.3 to 0.5 grams of carb to a biscotti.

PREPARATION TIME: 35 minutes. BAKING TIME (IN TWO STAGES): 65 minutes. SERVING SIZE: 1 biscotti. AMOUNT PER SERVING: 1.6 grams of carb, 1.9 grams of protein. NUMBER OF SERVINGS: 45 to 50.

		CHO (g)	PRO (g)
4	ounces cream cheese, soft	3.2	8.4
4	tablespoons butter (½ stick), soft	0	0
4	egg yolks	1.2	11.2
16	packets Splenda sugar substitute	16.0	0
3	teaspoons vanilla	1.5	0
¼	teaspoon almond extract	0.1	0
1	teaspoon grated lemon peel (or lemon extract)	0.1	0
¼	cup unbleached, all-purpose wheat (white) flour	23.0	3.0
¼	cup vital wheat gluten flour	5.6	26.0
1	teaspoon baking powder	1.2	0
1½	cups whole almond meal or blanched almond flour	18.0	36.0
	Total	*69.9*	*84.6*

Combine and beat the cream cheese, butter, and 2 egg yolks in the bowl of an electric mixer with a flat beater until thick, smooth, and creamy; do not underbeat. Add the other 2 egg yolks and beat for another minute. Add all of the remaining ingredients at slow speed or stirring by hand. Refrigerate the dough for about 30 minutes or until it can be handled without sticking.

Preheat oven to 300°F or 325°F.

Shape the dough in three rolls about 1¾ inches in diameter and about 12 inches long. Set the rolls on a nonstick, heavy-gauge metal cookie sheet and flatten them into bars about 2 inches wide and ¾ inch high. Bake for about 18 to 20 minutes or until golden (check early). Cool before slicing.

Set (or reduce) oven temperature to 225°F. To slice the small loaves, put them on a cutting board and slice each in about 15 pieces (use a sharp, serrated knife). Set pieces upright on the cookie sheet. Bake the biscotti until they have a light golden color, about 45 minutes (always check early—do not let them turn too dark). Allow the biscotti to cool, harden, and dry completely. Add the optional glaze once the cookies are hard and dry.

Variation: **Reduced-Carb Almond**   *(gluten-free)* **Biscotti**

Follow the Best Almond Biscotti recipe on page 258, but omit the wheat (white) flour and the vital wheat gluten flour. Add ½ cup soy protein powder and increase the whole almond meal to 1¾ cups. This reduces a biscotti to 1.0 gram of carb. The protein increase is minimal.

Variation: **Best Hazelnut Biscotti**

Follow the Best Almond Biscotti recipe on page 258, but omit the almond extract. Reduce the whole almond meal to ½ cup and add 1¼ cups ground, unblanched, natural hazelnuts. There is no significant change in carb and protein per cookie.

Chocolate Chip Cookies

If you miss chocolate chip cookies, try this one. A little white flour and brown sugar raise the carbs higher, but a small cookie still has only 1.6 grams of carb* and is divine.

PREPARATION TIME: 40 minutes. BAKING TIME: 12 to 16 minutes per batch.
SERVING SIZE: 1 cookie. AMOUNT PER SERVING: 1.6 grams of carb, 1.2 grams of protein. NUMBER OF SERVINGS: 75 to 80.

		CHO (g)	PRO (g)
4	egg yolks	1.2	11.2
3	tablespoons brown sugar lightly packed	36.0	0
15	packets Splenda sugar substitute	15.0	0
8	tablespoons butter (1 stick), soft	0	0
2	teaspoons vanilla extract	1.0	0
3	tablespoons unbleached, all-purpose wheat (white) flour	17.3	2.3
⅓	cup vital wheat gluten flour	7.5	34.7
2	tablespoons crude wheat bran	1.5	1.0
1	teaspoon baking powder	1.2	0
¾	cup whole almond meal	9.0	18.0
	trace salt	0	0
1½	ounces semisweet chocolate chips (scant ⅓ cup)	27.0	3.0
¾	cup chopped walnuts	6.0	20.7
	Total	*122.7*	*90.9*

Preheat oven to 300°F or 325°F about the time you take the dough from the fridge. Use two large, nonstick, heavy-gauge metal cookie sheets.

Put the egg yolks, brown sugar, and Splenda in the bowl of an electric mixer and beat until thick and creamy. Add all of the other ingredients except the chocolate chips and walnuts. Beat at slow speed until smooth. Stir in the walnuts and chocolate chips. Refrigerate dough for 1 hour or until firm enough to handle.

Shape balls about the size of medium grapes and put them on the cookie sheets (about 40 fit on a 13- by 18-inch sheet). Bake the cookies for about 12 to 16 minutes or until lightly browned. Cool. These cookies freeze well.

---

* This is the average carb count per cookie. The chocolate chips will have a somewhat uneven distribution; some cookies may be slightly higher (or lower) in carbs.

Sugar Cookies

A rich, flaky cookie with a delicious taste. It has a Sugar Glaze (page 275), but you can also use a Chocolate-Flavored Glaze (page 275). This cookie may become one of your favorites. If you want to save the cost of the icing (0.5 gram of carb), you can leave the cookies plain and merely increase the sweetness of the dough. Without icing, a cookie has 0.7 gram of carb, with icing, 1.2 grams of carb.

PREPARATION TIME: 50 minutes. BAKING TIME: 8 to 10 minutes per batch.
SERVING SIZE: 1 cookie (without icing). AMOUNT PER SERVING: 0.7 gram of carb, 0.9 gram of protein. NUMBER OF SERVINGS: 95 to 100.

		CHO (g)	PRO (g)
4	ounces cream cheese, soft	3.2	6.3
2	tablespoons butter (¼ stick), soft	0	0
4	egg yolks	1.2	11.2
12	packets Splenda sugar substitute*	12.0	0
2	teaspoons vanilla extract	1.0	0
2	teaspoons grated lemon peel (or lemon extract)	0.2	0
¼	cup unbleached, all-purpose wheat (white) flour	23.0	3.0
¼	cup vital wheat gluten flour	5.8	26.0
1	teaspoon baking powder	1.2	0
	trace of salt (shake or two)	0	0
1½	cups blanched almond flour	18.0	36.0
	Total	*65.6*	*82.5*

Combine the cream cheese, butter, and 2 egg yolks in the bowl of an electric mixer with a flat beater. Beat until thick, smooth, and creamy; do not underbeat. Add the other 2 egg yolks and beat for another minute. Stop the mixer. Add the remaining ingredients, then mix at slow speed or by hand. Refrigerate the dough for about 30 minutes or until it can be handled without sticking.

Preheat oven to 300°F or 325°F when you take the dough from the fridge. Use two large, nonstick, heavy-gauge metal cookie sheets.

Form balls the size of small grapes and put them on the cookie sheets. Allow room for expansion. About 24 cookies fit on a 13-by 18-inch cookie sheet. Flatten each cookie slightly with your fingertips. Next, rub a pinch of soy protein powder or soy flour on the contact surface of a smooth lid from a screw-top jar or a small flat-bottom glass. Press down firmly on each cookie. The cookies should expand to 2 or 2¼ inches. With a pastry brush, remove remnants of soy that may cling to the cookies. (Add soy to the contact surface as needed.)

Bake the cookies for 8 to 10 minutes (check early). Cookies should be barely golden with a slightly darker edge (avoid having the edge turn too dark). Apply Sugar Glaze (page 275) or Chocolate-Flavored Glaze (page 275), if desired, and allow to dry completely. These cookies are great keepers (even at room temperature). They also freeze well.

Variation: Ginger Snaps

Follow the recipe for Sugar Cookies on page 261, adding 1 table-spoon ground ginger, 1½ teaspoons ground cinnamon, ½ teaspoon ground nutmeg, and ¼ teaspoon ground cloves. Increase the packets of Splenda sugar substitute from 12 to 24. Increase the whole almond meal to 1¾ cups and omit the blanched almond meal. Each cookie, based on a count of 95, has 0.8 gram of carb.

---

* If you plan to make the cookies without a glaze, increase the Splenda sweetener to 22 packets for the recipe or adjust to taste. This raises the carb grams for a cookie to 0.8. A packet has 1.0 gram of carb.

The Lowest-Carb Cookies

These cookies are the lowest carb in this book. If you like to eat a big bunch of cookies at one session or have only a few carbs to splurge, these cookies will be lifesavers.

PREPARATION TIME: 30 to 35 minutes. BAKING TIME: 8 to 10 minutes per batch. SERVING SIZE: 1 cookie. AMOUNT PER SERVING: 0.5 gram of carb, 1.1 grams of protein. NUMBER OF SERVINGS: 95 to 100 cookies.

		CHO (g)	PRO (g)
4	ounces cream cheese, soft	3.2	6.3
3	tablespoons butter, soft	0	0
4	egg yolks	1.2	11.2
12	packets Splenda sugar substitute	12.0	0
2	teaspoons vanilla extract	1.0	0
2	teaspoons grated lemon peel (or lemon extract)	0.2	0
¼	cup crude wheat bran	3.0	2.0
⅔	cup soy protein powder	0	42.7
1	teaspoon baking powder	1.2	0
	trace of salt (shake or two)	0	0
1¾	cups whole almond meal	21.0	42.0
	Total	*42.8*	*104.2*

Combine the cream cheese, butter, and 2 egg yolks in the bowl of an electric mixer with a flat beater. Beat until thick, smooth, and creamy; do not underbeat. Add the other 2 egg yolks and beat for another minute. Stop the mixer. Add all of the remaining ingredients, then mix at slow speed or stir by hand. Refrigerate the dough for about 30 minutes or until it is firm enough to handle.

Preheat oven to 300°F or 325° about the time the dough is taken from the fridge.

Form balls the size of small grapes and put them on two nonstick, heavy-gauge metal cookie sheets. Allow room for expansion. About 24 cookies fit on a 13- by 18-inch cookie sheet. Flatten each cookie slightly with your fingertips. Next, rub a pinch of soy protein powder or soy flour on the contact surface of a smooth lid from a screw-top jar or a small flat-bottom glass. Press down firmly on each cookie. The cookies should expand to 2 or 2¼ inches. With a pastry brush, remove remnants of soy that may cling to the cookies. (Add soy to the contact surface as needed.)

Bake the cookies for 8 to 10 minutes (check early). Cookies should be light golden with a slightly darker edge (avoid having the edges turn too dark). These cookies are great keepers (even at room temperature). They also freeze well.

Coconut Macaroons

These macaroons are a bonanza for coconut lovers, much lower in carb than the traditional version. No matter how fine, run the coconut through the food processor. A commercial coconut macaroon of similar size has about 4.0 grams of carb; ours has 1.1 grams.

PREPARATION TIME: 40 minutes. BAKING TIME: 11 to 14 minutes per batch.
SERVING SIZE: 1 cookie. AMOUNT PER SERVING: 1.1 grams of carb, 0.7 gram of protein. NUMBER OF SERVINGS: 75.

		CHO (g)	PRO (g)
3	egg yolks	0.9	8.4
2	tablespoons brown sugar, lightly packed	24.0	0
4	tablespoons butter (½ stick), soft	0	0
1	egg	0.6	6.0
2	teaspoons vanilla extract	1.0	0
2	teaspoons grated lemon peel (or lemon extract)	0.2	0
18	packets Splenda sugar substitute	18.0	0
1	tablespoon vital wheat gluten flour	1.4	6.5
1	tablespoon stoneground whole-wheat flour	4.5	2.0
1½	teaspoons baking powder	1.2	0
	trace of salt (shake or two)	0	0
2½	cups finely ground, dried coconut (unsweetened)	19.0	16.0
½	cup whole almond meal	6.0	12.0
	Total	*77.4*	*50.9*

Preheat oven to 300°F to 325°F. (If you choose to refrigerate the dough for a while, preheat oven about the time you take the dough from the fridge.)

Put the egg yolks, brown sugar, and butter in the bowl of an electric mixer with a flat beater and beat until thick and creamy. Add the whole egg and beat for another minute. Add the vanilla extract, lemon peel (or extract), Splenda, vital wheat gluten flour, stoneground whole-wheat flour, baking powder, and salt. Beat just until mixed. By hand, fold in the coconut and almond meal.

Fill a small ice cream scoop (1 inch) with dough (level off bottom) and drop the dough on two nonstick, heavy-gauge metal cookie sheets. Leave space for some expansion. You can also refrigerate the dough for about 1 hour until it is no longer sticky and shape it into balls with your hands. Either way, flatten the cookies slightly with your fingertips and bake them for about 11 to 14 minutes or until they begin to turn light golden brown.

Hazelnut Nuggets

(gluten-free)

These hazelnut cookies are incredibly delicious and explode with hazelnut flavor. You can control the texture, making the cookies either chewy or crunchy, by the length of time you bake them. To get that great taste and texture, these cookies require a fairly large amount (for low-carb) of sugar. Although the sugar content is fairly high, the large amount of hazelnuts helps keep the overall carb count reasonably low.

PREPARATION TIME: 45 minutes. BAKING TIME: 12 to 16 minutes per batch.
SERVING SIZE: 1 cookie. AMOUNT PER SERVING: 1.3 grams of carb, 0.9 gram of protein. NUMBER OF SERVINGS: 80 to 85.

		CHO (g)	PRO (g)
5	egg yolks	1.5	14.0
1	egg	0.6	3.5
¼	cup sugar	48.0	0
2	teaspoons vanilla extract	1.0	0
15	packets Splenda sugar substitute	15.0	0
1	tablespoon soy protein powder	0	4.0
1	tablespoon whey protein powder	0.8	5.0
	trace of salt (shake or two)	0	0
3	cups natural, unblanched, ground hazelnuts	32.4	44.4
	Total	*99.3*	*70.9*

Preheat oven to 300°F or 325°F. (If you decide to refrigerate the dough, preheat oven about the time you take the dough from the fridge.)

Put the egg yolks and egg in the bowl of an electric mixer with a flat beater and beat on high speed until thick and creamy. Gradually, by the tablespoon, approximately, add the sugar. Beat until very thick and creamy. Do not underbeat. Stop the mixer. Add the vanilla extract, Splenda, soy protein powder, whey protein powder, and salt. Mix on slow speed until combined. Remove the bowl from the mixer stand and gently fold in the hazelnuts about a cup at a time.

With a small ice cream or cookie scoop (1 inch), drop dough on two nonstick, heavy-gauge metal cookie sheets. The cookies do not need much space. You can also drop them on the cookie sheets with teaspoons (these cookies will not be smooth). Or refrigerate the dough for 30 minutes or until no longer sticky. Shape by hand in balls the size of medium grapes. Flatten all cookies lightly with your fingertips before baking. For chewy cookies, bake about 12 minutes; they should show almost no color. For crunchy cookies, bake about 16 minutes or until golden. Cool. Freeze surplus cookies soon after baking if you want to preserve a chewy texture.

Black Soybean Spice Cookies

Black bean cookies or cakes are a delightful Chinese treat. Real black beans, which are normally used, are high in carbs, but mashed black soybeans make a pretty good substitute. These cookies are lightly spiced, chewy, and easy to make. They are great for lunch boxes.

PREPARATION TIME: 30 to 40 minutes. BAKING TIME: 15 to 18 minutes per batch.

SERVING SIZE: 1 cookie. AMOUNT PER SERVING: 1.2 grams of carb, 1.1 grams of protein. NUMBER OF SERVINGS: 80 to 85.

		CHO (g)	PRO (g)
3	egg yolks	0.9	8.4
3	tablespoons brown sugar, lightly packed	36.0	0
6	tablespoons butter (¾ stick), soft	0	0
15	packets Splenda	15.0	0
⅔	cup mashed black soybeans	4.3	9.2
1½	teaspoons ground cinnamon	1.1	0
¼	teaspoon ground cloves	0.3	0
1½	teaspoons baking powder	1.2	0
	trace of salt (shake or two, optional)	0	0
¼	cup stoneground whole-wheat flour	18.1	4.0
¼	cup vital wheat gluten flour	5.6	26.0
¾	cup whole almond meal	9.0	18.0
¾	cup chopped black walnuts	6.0	21.0
	Total	*97.5*	*86.6*

Put the egg yolks and brown sugar in the bowl of an electric mixer with a flat beater and beat on high speed until thick and creamy. Stop mixer. Add all of the other ingredients except the walnuts. Beat at slow speed until smooth. Stir in the walnuts by hand.

Refrigerate the dough for about 1 hour or until firm enough to handle. Preheat oven to 300°F to 325°F. Shape the dough into balls the size of medium-size grapes and drop on two nonstick, heavy-gauge metal cookie sheets. Flatten all cookies lightly with your fingertips. Bake cookies for about 15 to 18 minutes or until lightly browned. Cool. To keep cookies chewy, freeze. They also taste great if they get a little crisp.

Variation: Black Soybean Tea Cakes

These are delicious, soft, chewy, small cakes. Follow the directions for making the cookies. When you shape the cakes, make them walnut size. You should end up with 28 cakes. Shape them as you would the cookies by flattening them with your fingertips. Bake them for an extra 2 minutes. Each tea cake has 3.5 grams of carb and 3.1 grams of protein. You can also add ¼ cup raisins to the dough. It adds 0.9 gram of carb per tea cake.

Pumpkin Spice Cookies

A fabulous cookie—sure to test your self-discipline. Despite some high-carb ingredients, a cookie has only 1.6 grams of carb.

PREPARATION TIME: 30 to 40 minutes. BAKING TIME: 15 to 18 minutes per batch.

SERVING SIZE: 1 cookie. AMOUNT PER SERVING: 1.6 grams of carb, 1.0 gram of protein. NUMBER OF SERVINGS: 80 cookies.

		CHO (g)	PRO (g)
3	tablespoons brown sugar	36.0	0
3	egg yolks	0.9	8.4
6	tablespoons butter (¾ stick), soft	0	0
15	Splenda sugar substitute packets	15.0	0
½	cup canned pumpkin	4.0	2.0
1½	teaspoons ground cinnamon	1.1	0
½	teaspoon ground nutmeg	0.6	0
¼	teaspoon ground cloves	0.3	0
1	teaspoon baking powder	1.2	0
	trace of salt (shake or two)	0	0
¼	cup stoneground whole-wheat flour	18.1	4.0
¼	cup vital wheat gluten flour	5.6	26.0
¾	cup whole almond meal	9.0	18.0
¼	cup raisins	26.0	1.0
¾	cup chopped black walnuts	6.0	20.7
	Total	*123.8*	*80.1*

Put the egg yolks and sugar in the bowl of an electric mixer with a flat beater and beat until thick and creamy. Stop mixer. Add all of the other ingredients except the walnuts and raisins. Beat at slow speed until smooth. Stir in the walnuts and raisins by hand. Refrigerate the dough for 1 hour or until firm enough to handle.

Preheat oven to 300°F to 325°F when you take the dough from the fridge.

Shape the dough into balls the size of medium-size grapes. Flatten all cookies lightly with your fingertips before baking. Bake for about 15 to 18 minutes or until lightly browned. Cool. To keep cookies chewy, freeze. They also taste great if they get a little crisp.

Scrumptious Low-Carb Cheesecake

You will find this to be one of the best-tasting cheesecakes you have ever had. For a crust, choose the Cookie/Pecan Crust on page 292 or the gluten-free Waffle/Pecan Crust on page 292. Remember that these carb and protein counts are for the filling only.

PREPARATION TIME (CHEESECAKE FILLING ONLY): 20 minutes. BAKING TIME: 45 to 55 minutes.

SERVING SIZE (FILLING ONLY): 1 piece. AMOUNT PER SERVING: 3.9 grams of carb, 5.3 grams of protein. NUMBER OF SERVINGS: 12.

		CHO (g)	PRO (g)
CHEESECAKE FILLING			
20	ounces cream cheese, soft	16.0	42.0
4	egg yolks	1.2	11.2
2	teaspoons lemon juice (or to taste)	0.9	0
2	teaspoons vanilla extract	1.0	0
20	packets Splenda sugar substitute	20.0	0
1	tablespoon stoneground whole-wheat flour	4.5	1.0
⅓	cup sour cream	2.7	2.1
2	egg whites	0.6	7.0
	Total	*46.9*	*63.3*

Prepare a crust of your choice. Butter the bottom and sides of an 8- or 9- inch springform pan and follow crust directions. (Because low-carb ingredients, such as those used in cookies or waffles, tend to brown or darken more quickly, it is best to use a heavy-gauge metal springform pan; see "Mail-Order Resources.")

Preheat oven to 300°F or 325°F.

Put the cream cheese and 2 egg yolks in the bowl of an electric mixer with a flat beater. Beat just until smooth and all cream cheese lumps are gone. Add the other 2 egg yolks and beat until mixed. On slow speed, combine the rest of the ingredients except the egg whites just until mixed.

Beat the egg whites until firm but not stiff; fold gently into the batter with a spatula. Pour the batter into the springform pan. Bake for about 45 to 55 minutes until the cake is light golden. Turn oven off. Do not remove the cheesecake. Keep door slightly ajar and allow cake to cool in the oven for about an hour. Refrigerate. Cheesecakes always shrink a little in the center. This one shrinks just mildly. Serve plain or with dribbles of Cranberry Sauce (page 299) or fresh fruit. This cheesecake will last, covered, for several days in the fridge. It also freezes. (If you like, cut the cheesecake in serving pieces before freezing; then you can easily remove what you want.) Thaw in fridge.

Coconut Layer Cake

A great cake to serve on virtually any occasion. Try to buy the finest grind of coconut you can; look for "macaroon coconut." No matter how fine, run the coconut through the food processor. Frost cake with Creamy Vanilla Frosting (page 277) or Velvety Chocolate Frosting (page 278). You can also use heavy cream (about ⅔ cup), whipped, sweetened to taste, and flavored with a hint of coconut extract. Remember that these carb and protein counts are for the cake only.

PREPARATION TIME (CAKE ONLY): 15 minutes. BAKING TIME: 35 to 40 minutes.

SERVING SIZE: 1 slice (cake only). AMOUNT PER SERVING: 4.8 grams of carb, 7.5 grams of protein. NUMBER OF SERVINGS: 12.

		CHO (g)	PRO (g)
4	ounces cream cheese, soft	3.2	8.4
2	tablespoons butter (¼ stick), soft	0	0
5	eggs, separated	3.0	30.0
¼	cup light or heavy cream	1.6	1.2
¼	cup vital wheat gluten flour	5.6	26.0
½	cup whole almond meal	6.0	12.0
1	teaspoon baking powder	1.2	0
	trace of salt (one or two light shakes)	0	0
2	teaspoons vanilla extract	1.0	0
1	teaspoon coconut extract (optional)	0.2	0
20	packets Splenda sugar substitute	20.0	0
2	cups finely ground, dried coconut (unsweetened)	16.0	12.8
	Total	*57.8*	*90.4*

Preheat oven to 325°F. Butter an 8- or 9-inch nonstick, heavy-gauge metal springform pan.

Beat the cream cheese, butter, and 2 egg yolks in the bowl of an electric mixer with a flat beater until thick and creamy. Add the other 3 egg yolks and beat again. Add all of the other ingredients except the coconut and the egg whites at low speed until mixed. Fold in the coconut flakes with a spatula.

Beat the 5 egg whites until firm but not stiff and fold into the batter with a spatula. Distribute the batter evenly in the springform pan and bake for 35 to 40 minutes or until golden brown and a knife inserted in the center comes out clean (check early). Cool. Slice the cake in half horizontally and frost the two layers as desired.

Variation: Hazelnut Cake

Follow the directions for making Coconut Layer Cake on page 270, but reduce the whole almond meal to ¼ cup. Omit the coconut. Add 2 cups natural, ground, unblanched hazelnuts. Carb count for entire cake is 60.4 grams; protein is 101.2 grams. You can also bake this cake in three heavy-gauge metal mini loaf pans (3 by 6 inches) and glaze the small cakes with an optional Lemon Sugar Glaze (page 276.) Total carbs, minus glaze, are 64.5 grams. Total protein is 109.1 grams. Bake the loaves for about 35 to 40 minutes or until done. If you cut 30 slices, a slice has 2.0 grams of carb and 3.4 grams of protein. The optional glaze adds about 1.0 gram of carb per slice. The cake freezes well.

Rich Low-Carb Pound Cake

This tastes great and is quick and easy to make. For best results, bake the cake in three miniloaf pans (3 by 6 inches). If you cut each loaf (of three) in 10 thick slices, each slice will have 3.3 grams of carb. A commercial pound cake slice has 16.0 grams of carb.

PREPARATION TIME: 15 minutes. BAKING TIME: 40 to 50 minutes.
SERVING SIZE: 1 slice. AMOUNT PER SERVING: 2.8 grams of carb, 3.9 grams of protein. NUMBER OF SERVINGS: 30.

		CHO (g)	PRO (g)
4	ounces cream cheese, soft	3.2	8.4
8	tablespoons butter, soft (1 stick)	0	0
5	eggs, separated	3.0	30.0
¼	cup light or heavy cream	1.6	1.2
½	cup stoneground whole-wheat flour	36.2	8.0
¼	cup vital wheat gluten flour	5.6	26.0
½	cup soy protein powder	0	32.0
1	teaspoon baking powder	1.2	0
	trace of salt (two or three light shakes)	0	0
3	teaspoons vanilla extract	1.5	0
2	teaspoons grated lemon peel		
	(or lemon extract)	0.2	0
24	packets Splenda sugar substitute	24.0	0
½	cup whole almond meal	6.0	12.0
	Total	82.5	117.6

Preheat oven to 325°F. Lightly grease three small, nonstick, heavy-gauge metal miniloaf pans (3 by 6 inches).

Put the cream cheese, butter, and 2 egg yolks in the bowl of an electric mixer with a flat beater and beat until thick and creamy. Add the other 3 egg yolks and beat. Add all of the other ingredients except the almond meal and the egg whites and mix at low speed. Add the almond meal last and mix in gently.

Beat the egg whites until firm but not stiff and fold carefully into the batter. Distribute batter evenly in the miniloaf pans and bake for 40 to 50 minutes or until golden brown and a knife inserted in the center comes out clean. Cool completely before slicing. The cake freezes well.

Variation: Fruity Pound Cake

Add 1 cup of your favorite fruit to the batter before baking. Blueberries, strawberries, blackberries, and raspberries all work wonderfully.

Poppy Seed Cake

If you like poppy seeds, this cake will delight you. If you cut each loaf (of three) into 10 thick slices, each slice will have 3.3 grams of carb. (You can add an optional Lemon Sugar Glaze, page 276. The glaze will add 1.1 grams of carb to each slice.) The cake freezes well.

PREPARATION TIME: 30 minutes. BAKING TIME: 30 to 50 minutes depending on the size of pans.

SERVING SIZE: 1 slice. AMOUNT PER SERVING: 3.3 grams of carb, 3.9 grams of protein. NUMBER OF SERVINGS: 30.

		CHO (g)	PRO (g)
3	tablespoons poppy seeds	3.6	5.0
½	cup heavy cream	3.2	2.4
4	ounces cream cheese, soft	3.2	8.4
2	tablespoons butter (¼ of a stick), soft	0	0
5	eggs, separated	3.0	30.0
½	cup stoneground whole-wheat flour	36.2	8.0
¼	cup vital wheat gluten flour	5.6	26.0
1	teaspoon baking powder	1.2	0
	trace of salt (two or three light shakes)	0	0
2	teaspoons vanilla extract	1.0	0
2	teaspoons grated lemon peel (or lemon extract)	0.2	0
24	packets Splenda sugar substitute	24.0	0
1½	cups whole almond meal	18.0	36.0
	Total	*99.2*	*115.8*

Soak poppy seeds overnight in cream in the fridge. When ready to bake, simmer the poppy seeds in the cream for about 10 minutes, in a small saucepan over very low heat, uncovered. Stir often. Cool before adding to the cake batter.

Preheat oven to 325°F. Lightly grease three nonstick, heavy-gauge metal mini loaf pans. Put a narrow strip of waxed paper in each and allow to overhang on top of pan about 2 inches on each end so you can pick up cake easily when it is baked.

Put the cream cheese, butter, and 2 egg yolks in the bowl of an electric mixer with a flat beater and beat until thick and creamy. Add the other 3 egg yolks and beat again (do not underbeat). Add the poppy seed–cream mixture, wheat (white) flour, vital wheat gluten flour, baking powder, salt, vanilla extract, lemon peel (or extract), and Splenda sugar substitute. Mix together at low speed. Add the almond meal at low speed.

Beat the egg whites until firm but not stiff and fold gently into the batter with a spatula. Distribute the batter evenly in the mini loaf pans and bake for 40 to 50 minutes or until golden brown (reduce baking time to about 30 or 35 minutes if you use smaller pans).

If you want to glaze the cake, prepare the Lemon Sugar Glaze (page 276) while the cake is baking. Brush the glaze thinly over the hot or warm loaves. Allow the loaves to cool completely and the glaze to harden before slicing. A slice (based on 30) will have 4.4 grams of carb.

Sugar Glaze

This incredible icing is made from egg white, powdered sugar, and vanilla. A miniscule amount delivers a small but potent dose of sweetness. Be sure to be sparing in your portions. The icing is easy to whip up and can be kept for a couple of weeks or longer in the fridge. Keep covered and stir before using. You can make the recipe with raw egg white or sterilized (homogenized) egg white, available in many supermarkets.

PREPARATION TIME: 5 minutes.
SERVING SIZE: icing for 1 cookie. AMOUNT PER SERVING: 0.5 gram of carb, no
   protein. NUMBER OF SERVINGS: 280.

	CHO (g)	PRO (g)
1 egg white (or 3 tablespoons sterilized egg white)	0.3	3.5
1 cup powdered sugar (unsifted)	128.0	0
3 teaspoons vanilla extract	1.5	0
Total	*129.8*	*3.5*

Put the egg white and powdered sugar in the bowl of your electric mixer and beat on high speed until the sugar is absorbed and the mixture thickens a bit; scrape sides of bowl as needed. Mix in the vanilla extract. Apply icing with the tip of a knife or a small brush. The icing dries quickly, particularly over freshly baked cookies, rolls, and so forth. Store unused frosting, covered, in the fridge. Always stir well before using.

Variation: Chocolate-Flavored Glaze

Follow the directions for making Sugar Glaze above, but reduce the powdered sugar to ¾ cup. Add 2 tablespoons of good-quality, unsweetened cocoa to the mixture. Use only 1 teaspoon vanilla extract and add 3 teaspoons chocolate extract.* Total carb count is 100.0 grams and protein is 3.5 grams. The glaze on one cookie has about 0.3 gram of carb and the protein is negligible. Use sparingly! (Keep extra glaze covered in fridge and stir before using.)

---

* Chocolate extract contains a small amount of red food coloring. Health experts consider this red color a carcinogen. If you want to avoid using the chocolate extract, increase the cocoa powder to 3 tablespoons. Add 3 to 4 teaspoons of water to the mix (to get the right consistency for spreading). A chocolate glaze made without the chocolate extract will not become quite as lustrous.

Lemon Sugar Glaze

This is a tangy, sweet glaze for cookies, rolls, cakes, cinnamon rolls, and other baked goods. It should have the consistency of very thin cream or even milk and will harden into a shiny, whisper-thin glaze. Because it is so sparingly applied, a little goes a long way; the carb count stays low. (Be sure to try this glaze on Magic Rolls, page 22. It turns them into fabulous sweet rolls. The rolls freeze well with the sugar glaze.)

PREPARATION TIME: 3 minutes

The amount is sufficient to cover 100 cookies at 0.3 gram of carb per cookie or two recipes (36 total) of Magic Rolls (page 22) at 0.9 gram of carb each.

	CHO (g)	PRO (g)
¼ cup powdered sugar (unsifted)	32.0	0
3 teaspoons lemon juice (or as desired)	1.3	0
Total	*33.3*	

In a small mixing bowl, combine the powdered sugar and lemon juice; stir until smooth. If needed, add water almost by the drop and stir after each addition. Dilute until the glaze is the desired consistency.

Creamy Vanilla Frosting

A rich frosting. It keeps refrigerated for a week or longer.

PREPARATION TIME: 15 minutes

SERVING SIZE: frosting and filling for 1 piece of cake. AMOUNT PER SERVING: 2.9 grams of carb, 1.0 gram of protein. NUMBER OF SERVINGS: 12.

		CHO (g)	PRO (g)
6	ounces cream cheese, soft	4.2	12.6
8	tablespoons butter (1 stick), soft	0	0
30	packets Splenda sugar substitute	30.0	0
3	teaspoons vanilla extract		
	(or as desired)	1.5	0
	Total	*35.7*	*12.6*

In the bowl of an electric mixer with a flat beater, beat the cream cheese and butter until the mixture is creamy, fluffy, and free of all cream cheese lumps. Beat in the Splenda and vanilla extract.

Velvety Chocolate Frosting

A rich, smooth frosting that is a perfect finish for a cake. Use as filling and/or frosting. It keeps refrigerated for a week or longer.

PREPARATION TIME: 15 minutes.
SERVING SIZE: frosting and filling for 1 slice of cake. AMOUNT PER SERVING: 3.2 grams of carb, 0.8 gram of protein. NUMBER OF SERVINGS: 16.

		CHO (g)	PRO (g)
2	ounces good-quality unsweetened chocolate	8.0	3.6
6	tablespoons butter (¾ stick), soft	0	0
¼	cup light or heavy cream	1.6	1.2
4	ounces cream cheese, soft	3.2	8.4
25	packets Splenda sugar substitute	25.0	0
1	teaspoon vanilla extract	0.5	0
	Total	*38.3*	*13.2*

Gently heat the chocolate, butter, and cream in the top of a double boiler until the chocolate is melted. Stir until smooth. Cool slightly.

In the bowl of an electric mixer with a flat beater, mix the cream cheese, Splenda, and vanilla extract until creamy. Add the chocolate mixture and beat well.

Dessert Waffles

(gluten-free)

These are light, crunchy, airy, sweet waffles that you can have ready for dessert almost at a moment's notice. They are sweeter than regular breakfast Waffles (page 53). Simply top waffles with sweetened whipped cream, fresh berries, or both. (Count all extra grams of carb.)

PREPARATION TIME: 10 minutes. COOKING TIME: 15 minutes.

SERVING SIZE: two 4-inch square waffles (or one 7- or 8-inch round waffle). AMOUNT PER SERVING: 6.7 grams of carb, 11.1 grams of protein. NUMBER OF SERVINGS: 5 or 6.

		CHO (g)	PRO (g)
4	ounces cream cheese, soft	3.2	8.4
1	egg	0.6	6.0
2	eggs, separated	1.2	12.0
20	packets Splenda sugar substitute	20.0	0
¼	cup soy protein powder	0	16.0
½	cup whole almond meal	6.0	12.0
¼	cup light or heavy cream	1.6	1.2
4	tablespoons melted butter (½ stick)	0	0
2	teaspoons vanilla extract	1.0	0
	Total	*33.6*	*55.6*

Preheat waffle iron.

Put the cream cheese and one egg in the bowl of an electric mixer with a flat beater and mix until smooth and creamy. Beat in the 2 egg yolks. At slow speed or by hand, mix in the remaining ingredients except the egg whites. Beat the egg whites separately until soft but firm peaks form. Fold them into the batter with a spatula.

Spoon the batter into the waffle iron. Low-carb waffles bake quickly. It will take from 3 to 5 minutes for a waffle (or waffles) to get done. Check early. It will not harm the waffles if you peek before they are ready.

Variation: Chocolate Dessert Waffles

Follow the directions for Dessert Waffles above, but increase the Splenda to 26 packets (or to taste). Melt 2 ounces of high-quality, unsweetened baking chocolate in the top of a double boiler. Cool slightly. Add the chocolate to the waffle batter before folding in the egg whites. This adds 14.0 grams of carb (total) to the waffles. A single serving has 9.5 grams of carb. The protein count remains virtually unchanged.

Jiffy Chocolate Whip   *(gluten-free)*

Make this quick dessert with Chocolate Dessert Waffles on page 279.
Though a snap to fix, it is not an instant dessert. It needs to ripen
overnight or longer.

PREPARATION TIME: 10 minutes. REFRIGERATION TIME: 24 hours or longer.
SERVING SIZE: ⅔ cup. AMOUNT PER SERVING: 11.0 grams of carb, 5.6 grams
of protein. NUMBER OF SERVINGS: 4.

		CHO (g)	PRO (g)
4	four-inch square or 2 round half servings of Chocolate Dessert Waffles (page 279)	13.4	22.2
1	cup heavy cream	6.4	4.8
15	packets Splenda sugar substitute	15.0	0
½	ounce semisweet chocolate, grated, optional	9.0	0.9
	Total	*43.8*	*27.9*

If the waffles come from the freezer, remove them ahead of time to
allow them to thaw and dry thoroughly. (If you are in a hurry, put the
waffles in a 300°F oven for 10 minutes or until dry.) Put the waffles in
a plastic bag and crush with a mallet or rolling pin. You can also pulse
them in the food processor.

Whip the cream until firm but not stiff. Stir in the Splenda. Reserve
about 4 tablespoons of the whipped cream. Fold the waffle crumbs
into the whipped cream and spoon in dessert glasses or bowls. Top
with a spoonful of whipped cream and sprinkle with the grated chocolate. Cover and chill for at least 24 hours.

Apple Brown Betty

This is an old, high-carb, comfort food favorite—apples and bread combined can pile up 50.0 grams of carbs per serving. This apple brown betty is every bit as good and has only 11.9 grams per serving. For the bread, you can use Best Whole-Wheat Bread (page 34) or either white or whole-wheat Magic Rolls (page 22). The directions are for Best Whole-Wheat Bread. If you want to use Magic Rolls, use five standard-size rolls for the recipe. The nutrition counts remain effectively unchanged. Cut the baking time for the cubed Magic Rolls in about half.

PREPARATION TIME: 30 minutes. TOTAL BAKING TIME: 37 to 50 minutes.
SERVING SIZE: ⅙ of total yield. AMOUNT PER SERVING: 11.7 grams of carb, 4.3 grams of protein. NUMBER OF SERVINGS: 6.

		CHO (g)	PRO (g)
4	ounces cubed Whole-Wheat Bread (page 34)	14.4	25.2
8	tablespoons butter (1 stick)	0	0
2½	cups peeled and sliced cooking apples	35.5	0.5
2	tablespoons lemon juice	1.3	0
18	packets Splenda sugar substitute	18.0	0
1	teaspoon ground cinnamon	0.6	0
⅛	teaspoon ground cloves	0.1	0
¼	teaspoon ground nutmeg	0.3	0
2	tablespoons butter (optional)	0	0
	Total	70.2	25.7

Preheat oven to 325°F. Butter a 12-inch square, nonstick, heavy-gauge metal baking pan or a medium-size ovenproof casserole dish.

Put the bread cubes on a nonstick, heavy-gauge metal cookie sheet and bake for about 12 to 15 minutes or until just barely browned. Put them in a medium-size mixing bowl.

Sprinkle apple slices with lemon juice to prevent browning.

Heat a heavy skillet on medium-low. Melt a half stick of butter in it. Add the apples to the skillet when the butter bubbles; do not brown. Cover and simmer the apples on low heat until soft, about 10–20 minutes, depending on the apples. Do not let apples brown. If skillet gets dry, add a little water to mixture. About halfway through, stir in the Splenda packets. When the apples are soft, remove skillet from the heat.

Melt 3 tablespoons of butter in the microwave or in a small saucepan. Stir in the cinnamon, cloves, nutmeg, and the other 9 Splenda packets. Pour this mixture over the baked bread cubes. Stir in quickly to cover the cubes as evenly as possible.

Put about half of the bread cubes in the bottom of the baking pan. Top with the apples. Put the remaining bread cubes on top. Dot with 1 tablespoon butter, if desired. Bake for about 25 to 35 minutes or until the top is lightly browned.

Serve warm with ice cream, fresh cream, or whipped cream. Count added carb and protein grams.

Variation: **Apple Brown Betty with Raisins**

For a special-occasion treat, add a few raisins to this dessert. Follow directions as given, but reduce the Splenda sugar substitute packets to 8 and do not add Splenda to the apples. When you put the layer of sautéed apples in the baking dish, sprinkle them evenly with 3 tablespoons of raisins. A serving, based on six, has 13.8 grams of carb.

Key Lime Pie

Key lime pie is exceptionally tasty. Key limes are hard to find, though. If you see them, buy some! A good substitute is bottled key lime juice. Use a prebaked Flaky Pastry Pie Crust (page 290) for this pie. This pie is also delicious made with regular limes or even lemons. Use the same amount of juice.

PREPARATION TIME (FILLING ONLY): 25 minutes (must be refrigerated for several hours or overnight).

SERVING SIZE (FILLING ONLY): 1 piece. AMOUNT PER SERVING: 6.1 grams of carb, 4.9 grams of protein. NUMBER OF SERVINGS: 8.

		CHO (g)	PRO (g)
1	prebaked Flaky Pastry Pie Crust (page 290)	25.8	31.8
FILLING			
1	packet unflavored gelatin	0	6.0
½	cup key lime juice	11.2	0
20	packets Splenda sugar substitute	18.0	0
1½	cups heavy cream	9.6	7.2
12	ounces cream cheese, soft	9.6	26.2
	Total	*74.2*	*71.2*

Soak the gelatin in ¼ cup cold water. Meanwhile, in a small saucepan, heat the key lime juice on medium-low; do not boil. Add the soaked gelatin mix to the hot lime juice. Take it from the heat and stir in the gelatin until it is dissolved (about 1 minute). Mix in the Splenda. Put the saucepan in the fridge while you whip the cream cheese and cream (use a trivet). Never allow it to solidify or the pie will have little gelatin chunks.

Beat the cream until quite firm but not stiff. Set aside.

In the bowl of an electric mixer with a flat beater, mix the cream cheese until smooth and fluffy; it should be completely free of lumps. Remove the lime-gelatin mix from the fridge. It will still be thin. Whisk the juice mix for a moment. Dribble about ¼ cup into the cream cheese and beat well. Add the rest slowly and beat again.

Fold the whipped cream into the mixture. Taste for sweetness. The pie will be quite soft but firm enough to pile into a pie shell. (The carbs for the pie shell of your choice must be added to the count per serving.) Cover loosely and refrigerate pie for at least 3 hours or overnight. If you like, serve with a dribble of Cranberry Sauce (page 299; count added carbs).

Chocolate Orange Crème Pie

This dessert just melts in your mouth with lovely flavors and a divine, creamy texture. It needs neither baking nor gelatin to hold it together. Just melt some chocolate, combine it with cream cheese, whipped cream, sweetener, and orange flavor—you're done. Serve this dessert as is in a prebaked Flaky Pastry Pie Crust (page 290). You can also skip the crust and serve the dessert in glasses or bowls. The pie keeps, covered, for a few days in the fridge.

PREPARATION TIME (WITHOUT PIE CRUST): 20 minutes.

SERVING SIZE: 1 piece. AMOUNT PER SERVING: 8.8 grams of carb, 5.1 grams of protein. NUMBER OF SERVINGS: 12.

		CHO (g)	PRO (g)
1	prebaked Flaky Pastry Pie Crust (page 00)	25.8	31.8
3	ounces semisweet chocolate	54.0	6.0
2	tablespoons butter (¼ stick)	0	0
2	teaspoons orange extract or as desired*	1.0	0
8	ounces cream cheese, soft	6.4	16.8
1¼	cups heavy cream	8.0	6.0
8	packets Splenda sugar substitute	8.0	0
2	teaspoons semisweet, grated chocolate	2.5	0.4
	Total	*105.7*	*61.0*

Set aside one Flaky Pastry Pie Crust (page 290).

Gently melt the chocolate and butter in the top of a double boiler. Mix in the orange extract. Cool this mixture. If you are in a hurry, put it in the fridge for a few minutes.

Put the cream cheese in the bowl of an electric mixer with a flat beater and mix until smooth and creamy. Make sure there are no cream cheese lumps.

Beat the heavy cream until fairly stiff (a little more so than you would normally).

Add a small amount of the chocolate mixture (about 2 tablespoons) to the cream cheese and beat well. Stir in the rest of the chocolate slowly, until blended. Add the Splenda. Taste the mixture to check for orange flavor. If necessary, add more extract. Fold in the whipped cream with a spatula and pour into the pie shell. Dust the top with the grated chocolate.

* Orange extracts vary in intensity by brand; they also may lose some flavor after sitting on the shelf for a while (once opened).

Creamy Berry Pie

A dessert that is as easy to make as it is delicious—just mix lightly crushed berries with whipped cream. You can alter the proportion of berries, even add different kinds of fruit, if you like (just keep track of changes in carbs). In a pinch, this makes a nice dessert even without the pie crust. Serve in dessert glasses or bowls. Deduct 3.2 grams of carb and 4.0 grams of protein per serving.

PREPARATION TIME (WITHOUT PIE CRUST): 20 minutes. Must be refrigerated for 3 or more hours.

SERVING SIZE: 1 piece. AMOUNT PER SERVING: 9.3 grams of carb, 5.5 grams of protein. NUMBER OF SERVINGS: 8.

		CHO (g)	PRO (g)
1	prebaked Flaky Pastry Pie Crust (page 290)	25.8	31.8
1	packet gelatin	0	6.0
2	cups sliced strawberries	15.4	2.0
2	cups raspberries	11.6	1.2
2	tablespoons lemon juice	2.6	0
15	packets Splenda sugar substitute	15.0	0
⅔	cup heavy cream	4.3	3.2
	Total	*74.7*	*44.2*

Set aside a Flaky Pastry Pie Crust (page 290).

Soak the gelatin in 2 tablespoons of cold water.

Lightly crush the strawberries and raspberries (best done with a fork); put them in a medium-size mixing bowl. Save a few uncrushed berries for garnishing.

In a small saucepan, heat 2 tablespoons water and lemon juice. Do not boil. Add the soaked gelatin and stir until completely dissolved, about 1 minute. Remove from heat. Add the Splenda sugar substitute. Stir. Cool for a few minutes. Stir this sauce into the berries. Put the berries in the fridge while you whip the cream.

Whip the cream until quite firm but not totally stiff. Gently fold the whipped cream into the crushed berries with a spatula. Spoon the dessert into the pie shell or individual dessert dishes. Cover loosely and chill for 3 hours or overnight. Decorate with fresh berries (count any extra carb grams if you do).

Low-Carb Peach Cobbler

This cobbler is another dessert you can fix in a hurry. It is incredibly tasty and will be wildly popular. All fruit in these cobblers must go in the bottom of the baking pan. Use ripe, fresh peaches.

PREPARATION TIME: 20 minutes. BAKING TIME: 25 to 35 minutes.

SERVING SIZE: ⅛ total yield. AMOUNT PER SERVING: 9.2 grams of carb, 5.7 grams of protein. NUMBER OF SERVINGS: 8.

		CHO (g)	PRO (g)
2	cups freshly sliced peaches	30.0	0
4	packets Splenda sugar substitute*	4.0	0
1	tablespoon butter (optional)	0	0
BATTER			
3	ounces cream cheese, soft	2.4	6.3
1	tablespoon butter, soft	0	0
4	eggs, separated	1.2	24.0
⅓	cup light or heavy cream	2.1	1.6
2	teaspoons vanilla extract	1.0	0
¼	cup stoneground whole-wheat flour	18.1	3.0
2	tablespoons soy protein powder	0	8.0
2	tablespoons whole almond meal	1.5	3.0
1	teaspoon baking powder	1.2	0
12	packets Splenda sugar substitute	12.0	0
	trace of salt (two or three light shakes)	0	0
	Total	*73.5*	*45.9*

Preheat oven to 350°F. Butter an 8- by 8-inch or 9- by 12-inch ovenproof glass baking dish or a nonstick baking pan.

Lay the peaches evenly over the bottom of the baking dish. Sprinkle 4 packets of Splenda over the peaches. Dot with 1 tablespoon butter (optional).

Prepare the batter by beating the cream cheese, butter, and 1 egg yolk in the bowl of an electric mixer with a flat beater; beat until thick and creamy (no cream cheese lumps). Add the 3 other egg yolks and beat briefly again. Mix in the cream and vanilla extract. Add the remaining ingredients except the egg whites and stir just until mixed.

Beat the egg whites until firm but not stiff and fold or stir into the batter (this batter is a bit on the firm side). Spread the batter over the peaches and bake for about 25 to 35 minutes or until golden and done. Serve hot or cold.

Variation: Low-Carb Rhubarb Cobbler

Follow the directions for making Peach Cobbler on page 286, but omit the peaches. Substitute 3 cups of freshly chopped rhubarb. Total carbs for the rhubarb are only 10.0 grams. However, you need to increase the Splenda sugar substitute to 15 packets. A piece of rhubarb cobbler (based on 8 servings) has 7.6 grams of carb.

Variation: Low-Carb Apple Cobbler

Apples work nicely for this dessert if you cook them first. You can probably get by with 3 cups of peeled and sliced apples. That adds 42 grams of carb. Cook the sliced apples in a skillet in 2 tablespoons melted butter until tender and put them in the bottom of the baking dish. A piece of cobbler (based on 8 servings) has 10.2 grams of carb.

Variation: Low-Carb Strawberry Shortcake

This cobbler batter is light and airy. It makes eight great little short-cakes. Follow the directions for making the batter. Thoroughly butter individual 3-inch nonstick baking pans or use ramekins. Run a 1-inch strip of waxed paper across the bottom and up the sides, to help remove shortcakes that may stick a little. Distribute the batter evenly. These cakes are best used the day they are baked, but you can freeze them. Each shortcake has 4.9 grams of carb and 5.7 grams of protein. (Leave out the sweetener and you get 2.5 grams of carb each.) Pile strawberries and whipped cream on top. Count the extra carb grams.

Best Pumpkin Pie

Good news! Pumpkin pie can be on again for Thanksgiving and other celebrations. The main ingredient for pumpkin pie—pumpkin—is wonderfully low-carb (and high in fiber—5.0 grams in ½ cup). But to get a superb pie, the pumpkin needs a little pump-up from a dash of brown sugar. You know what that does to carb counts! Still, the carb count is low compared to commercial or regular homemade pies, which carry as much as 39.0 to 43.0 grams of carb in a piece (⅛ of a pie). Here it has 14.0 grams of carb, including the Flaky Pastry Pie Crust on page 290.

PREPARATION TIME (FILLING ONLY): 10 minutes. BAKING TIME: 45 to 55 minutes.

SERVING SIZE (FILLING ONLY): 1 piece. AMOUNT PER SERVING: 10.8 grams of carb, 3.4 grams of protein. NUMBER OF SERVINGS: 8.

		CHO (g)	PRO (g)
1	prebaked Flaky Pastry Pie Crust (page 290)	25.8	31.8
PUMPKIN PIE FILLING			
3	eggs	1.8	18.0
¼	cup brown sugar, lightly packed	48.0	0
15	packets Splenda sugar substitute	13.0	0
1	tablespoon ground cinnamon	2.1	0
¼	teaspoon ground cloves	1.0	0
½	teaspoon ground nutmeg	0.5	0
½	teaspoon ginger	0.6	0
	trace of salt (shake or two)	0	0
1½	cups canned pumpkin	12.0	3.3
1¼	cups heavy cream	8.0	6.0
	Total	*112.8*	*59.1*

Preheat oven to 325°F. Set aside one baked Flaky Pastry Pie Crust (page 290). Tear off two pieces of aluminum foil, each 12 by 13 inches.

Lightly beat together by hand eggs, sweeteners, spices, salt. Add the pumpkin and cream. Beat until just mixed. Pour the mixture into the pie shell.

Arrange the foil pieces crosswise and set the pie in the center. Turn up the foil and shape it around the outer edge of the pie to cover the exposed, fluted crust. Bake the pie for 45 to 55 minutes or until done (a knife inserted in the center should come out clean). Serve warm or cold. It will keep, covered, for 3 to 4 days in the fridge. Serve with a dollop of whipped cream if you like.

Apple Pie

You need a lot of apples for making apple pie. So no matter what you do, it's never going to be terrifically low-carb. The apples alone—based on 4 cups per pie—run up 7.1 grams of carb for 1 piece of pie—and that's without sugar! Still, if you crave a piece of apple pie now and then, this won't let you down. Bake the pie in the Flaky Pastry Pie Crust (page 290). It's a single shell and it adds 3.2 grams of carb to a serving.

PREPARATION TIME (FILLING ONLY): 20 minutes. BAKING TIME: 40 minutes.
SERVING SIZE (FILLING ONLY): 1 piece. AMOUNT PER SERVING: 11.2 grams of
carb, 1.7 grams of protein. NUMBER OF SERVINGS: 8.

		CHO (g)	PRO (g)
1	prebaked Flaky Pastry Pie Crust	25.8	31.8
FILLING			
4	cups peeled and thinly sliced cooking apples	56.8	0
1	tablespoon lemon juice	1.3	0
1	egg	0.6	6.0
2	egg yolks	0.9	5.6
20	packets Splenda sugar substitute	20.0	0
2	tablespoons stoneground whole-wheat flour	9.1	2.0
4	tablespoons butter (½ stick), soft (optional)	0	0
1	teaspoon ground cinnamon (optional)	0.6	0
	Total	*115.1*	*45.4*

Preheat oven to 325°F when you are ready to bake the pie. Have ready one Flaky Pastry Pie Crust (page 290). Tear off 2 pieces of aluminum foil, each 12 by 13 inches.

Sprinkle lemon juice over apples to prevent browning.

Lightly whisk the egg and egg yolks together. Combine the Splenda, flour, and spices. Add this mixutre to the eggs and whisk until dispersed. Pour the mixture over the apples, coating apples well. Fill the pie shell with the mixture and dot with the optional butter.

Arrange the foil pieces crosswise and set the pie in the center. Turn up the foil and shape it around the outer edge of the pie pan to cover the exposed, fluted crust. Bake the pie for 40 minutes or until the apples are done. Cool. Serve plain or with cheese or with a dollop of whipped cream, if desired. Count any added carbs. This pie will keep in the fridge, covered, for several days.

Flaky Pastry Pie Crust

This recipe makes a single, delicious, flaky pastry crust. You can have a crust ready to pop in the oven in 10 minutes. You can use it pre-baked, even when you bake it again with a filling in it. It keeps the bottom from getting soggy. This dough is easy to roll out.

PREPARATION TIME: 10 minutes. BAKING TIME (PREBAKED SHELL): 20 to 25 minutes.

SERVING SIZE (PIE CRUST ONLY): 1 piece. AMOUNT PER SERVING: 3.2 grams of carb, 4.0 grams of protein. NUMBER OF SERVINGS: 8.

	CHO (g)	PRO (g)
2 tablespoons vital wheat gluten flour	2.8	13.0
¼ cup stoneground whole-wheat flour	18.1	4.0
⅓ cup whole almond meal	4.0	8.0
2 tablespoons butter (¼ stick), cold	0	0
½ teaspoon baking powder	0.6	0
pinch of salt (shake or two)	0	0
1 egg yolk	0.3	2.8
1 tablespoon soy protein powder for rolling out dough, or as needed	0	4.0
Total	*25.8*	*31.8*

Preheat oven to 300°F or 325°F. Use a nonstick, heavy-gauge metal 9-inch pie pan. Tear off two 12- by 13-inch pieces of aluminum foil or use a pie guard. (A pie guard covers the outside edge of a pie to keep the fluted edge from darkening prematurely as the pie bakes.)

Add the wheat gluten flour, stoneground whole-wheat flour, almond meal, baking powder, and salt to a medium-size mixing bowl and stir together. Cut in the butter. With the tips of your fingers, turn the mix into fine crumbs. In a small mixing bowl, lightly beat or stir together the egg yolk and 2 tablespoons cold water. Pour the liquid into the dry mix and stir with a fork until mostly absorbed. Use your hand for the rest. Form a smooth, pliable dough. (If all the dry mix is not absorbed, add a few drops of cold water, not more than ½ teaspoon at a time.)

Spread a bit of soy protein powder on a large cutting board and put a kitchen towel under the board so that it won't slide. Flatten the dough with your hand and continue with a rolling pin. Turn dough several times. Roll the piece slightly larger than the pie pan. Line the pan with it. Patch dough if needed. You can fold under the overhang and make a thick, fluted edge or you can cut some off and save a few carbs. Prick the bottom liberally all over with a fork or you will get air bubbles. If the pie crust is to be baked only once (as for Creamy Berry Pie, page 285), bake it without foil protection. If you will bake it again (as for Apple Pie, page 289), put the aluminum foil sheets crosswise under the pan and fold them lightly all over the fluted edge of the pie to keep it from burning.

Bake the shell for about 20 to 25 minutes or until light golden brown.

Cookie/Pecan Crust

This crust can be used as a tart crust; it is relatively low in carb and quite delicious. It is just a bunch of cookie crumbs! You can use any cookies from this cookbook, so never throw out dry cookies. The cookies are sweet, so no added sweetener is needed. This crust can be prebaked or partially prebaked, then baked with a topping (see Low-Carb Cheesecake on page 269, for example).

PREPARATION TIME: 10 minutes. BAKING TIME: 8 to 20 minutes.

SERVING SIZE (PIE CRUST ONLY): 1 piece. AMOUNT PER SERVING: 3.3 grams of carb, 3.6 grams of protein. NUMBER OF SERVINGS: 8.

	CHO (g)	PRO (g)
1 egg white	0.3	3.5
⅔ cup assorted cookie crumbs		
(about 18 cookies)	20.0	16.0
¾ cup roasted, crushed pecans*	6.0	9.0
2 tablespoons butter, melted (¼ stick)	0	0
Total	*26.3*	*28.5*

Preheat oven to 300°F. Lightly butter a 10-inch tart pan or a 9-inch nonstick, heavy-gauge metal springform pan or a regular pie pan.

Lightly beat the egg white. Mix together the cookie crumbs and pecans. Stir in the butter and egg white. Press this mixture into the bottom of the pan you are using.

To fully bake the crust, bake it for 15 to 20 minutes or until it begins to brown lightly. If you plan to bake a topping or filling in the pan, bake the crust for about 8 or 9 minutes and remove from oven before it darkens.

Variation: Waffle/Pecan Crust   *(gluten-free)*

Follow the recipe for Cookie/Pecan Crust on page 292, but replace the cookies with Basic Waffles (page 53) or Dessert Waffles (page 279). Use 2 dry 4-inch-square waffles or equivalent. Crush waffles in a plastic bag with a rolling pin (or do it in a food processor). Add 6 packets of Splenda sugar substitute to the crumbs unless using Dessert Waffles, in which case you can skip the added sweetener. Carb and protein content of this crust is comparable to the Cookie/Pecan Crust.

---

* To roast the pecans, preheat oven to 325°F. Put the pecans in a shallow baking pan and roast for 15 to 20 minutes. Check early. Pecans tend to scorch quickly. Cool the nuts and crush in a food processor by pulsing briefly.

Basic Baked Custard

*This is just one of many different ways of making a simple baked cus-
tard. If you already have your own favorite way of making custard,
stick with it, but use a low-carb sweetener. This custard calls for 2
cups of heavy cream, water, and 4 egg yolks. Although this recipe
makes servings for four, you can bake the filling custard in six small
ramekins instead. That is about ⅓ cup per person (finish it off with
some fresh fruit).*

PREPARATION TIME: 10 minutes. BAKING TIME: 30 minutes.
SERVING SIZE: ½ cup. AMOUNT PER SERVING: 5.5 grams of carb, 5.2 grams of
protein. NUMBER OF SERVINGS: 4.

		CHO (g)	PRO (g)
1½	cups light or heavy cream	9.6	7.2
½	cup water	0	0
10	packets Splenda sugar substitute	10.0	0
2	teaspoons vanilla extract	1.0	0
	trace of salt (shake or two)	0	0
4	egg yolks	1.2	11.2
	Total	*21.8*	*18.4*

Preheat oven to 300°F. Have four to six small ovenproof ramekins
ready and butter them well. You can use any shape or size you wish.

Put all ingredients except egg yolks in a small saucepan. Heat on
medium-low heat, stirring occasionally with a wire whisk.

Put the egg yolks in a heavy glass jar. Beat the yolks with a wire
whisk until smooth. As the cream begins to heat and send off a little
steam, dribble some (about a tablespoon or so at a time) into the
yolks, constantly beating the yolks as you do. Repeat this a few more
times and add the rest of the cream to the eggs. For fussy palates,
strain the mix and return to the saucepan. Pour custard into baking
cups. Set the cups in a baking pan. Put the pan in the oven. Add about
½ inch of hot water to the pan (rather than fill it to the rim of the
ramekins). It will work just as well and is less of a hassle when you
want to move the pan.

Bake the custard for about 30 minutes. It should still be pale, but
shake like jelly. This time may vary depending on the size of your
pots. Cover the bowls and refrigerate.

Variation: Crème Brûlée

Follow the recipe for Basic Baked Custard (above). When you are
about ready to serve the chilled custard, preheat the broiler. Take

custards from the fridge and sprinkle 1 teaspoon of brown sugar over each. If the cups are broiler proof, put them in a broiling pan and put beneath the broiler (about 5 inches or so away) for about 90 seconds or until the sugar has melted. Serve immediately. It is much more convenient, though, to use a kitchen butane torch—worth getting if you like to make this dessert often. Each serving gains an extra 4.0 grams of carb.

Variation: Custard Cake

You can make this cake in 4 or 6 portions. (Directions are for 4.) However, these are large portions and some people may be satisfied with smaller ones. If you make 4 custard cakes, each will have 12.5 grams of carb; if you make 6 desserts, the carb count is 8.5 grams. Follow the recipe for Basic Baked Custard on page 293. Crush 6 cookies made from any recipe in this book into fine crumbs. Mix 2 tablespoons of instant, decaffeinated or regular coffee and 1 tablespoon of unsweetened cocoa powder with ½ cup boiling water; stir until dissolved. (Use ⅔ cup boiling water if you make 6 desserts.) Put 3 tablespoons of cookie crumbs in each bowl (2 tablespoons if you use 6 bowls) and dribble the coffee cocoa mix (evenly divided) over the crumbs. Do this before you make the custard. Carefully pour the custard over the soaked cookie crumbs. (Some will rise to the top during baking, but most stay at the bottom.) It gives the cake an intriguing look and texture. Turn the custard upside down when ready to serve. Top with a dollop of whipped cream (and count the extra carb grams).

Note: To dress up your custards, add fresh fruit in season. You can also use Rhubarb Sauce (page 299), Cranberry Sauce (page 299), or Uncooked Blueberry Sauce (page 300). Sprinkle a little nutmeg mixed with a packet of Splenda on top. Grate some chocolate and do the same. (Count any added carbs.)

Milk Chocolate Pecans

This is one of the best ways to satisfy a sweet tooth for an astonishingly small amount of carbs. A further saving grace is the good nutrition from the nuts when compared with ordinary sweets. The recipe is easy to make.

PREPARATION TIME: 15 to 20 minutes.

SERVING SIZE: 12 or 13 pecan halves. AMOUNT PER SERVING: 4.4 grams of carb, 2.6 grams of protein. NUMBER OF SERVINGS: 21.

		CHO (g)	PRO (g)
1	pound pecan halves	32.0	48.0
2	ounces milk chocolate	36.0	7.0
2	tablespoons butter (¼ stick)	0	0
2	tablespoons heavy cream	0.8	0.6
2	teaspoons vanilla extract	1.0	0
22	packets Splenda sugar substitute	22.0	0
	Total	*91.8*	*55.6*

Roast pecans. You can do this ahead of time and store the nuts for a few days until ready to use. Heat oven to 300°F or 325°F. Spread pecans in a shallow baking pan. Set them in the oven for about 20 to 25 minutes. Check early, pecans scorch easily. Do not let them brown. Cool.

Put the chocolate, butter, cream, vanilla extract, and Splenda in the top of a double boiler. Stir the mixture now and then while the chocolate melts gradually; it should be fully melted and smooth.

Put the roasted pecans in a large mixing bowl that will allow you to stir the nuts freely. When the chocolate mixture has melted, pour it over the pecans and stir to coat all of the nuts. Stir repeatedly; even distribution of the coating is important. Put the nuts in the fridge. Wait 5 minutes and stir again. Repeat twice more in 5-minute intervals. Avoid hardening the chocolate; it will form tiny lumps in the process. They do not hurt, but a fairly smooth coating looks nicer. Take the nuts from the fridge and put them on a cookie sheet or large tray. Use a fork to separate the nuts. They should form a single layer. A cool room is best; normal room temperature is okay, too. Within a few hours, the nuts will dry slightly and you can sample them. The nuts will dry fairly well within 24 hours. It will take a few days for them to dry completely. Meanwhile, cover them with paper towels or a light kitchen towel.

Variation: Milk Chocolate Pecan Balls

Follow the recipe for Milk Chocolate Pecans on page 295, but reduce the amount of pecans to 12 ounces. The nuts must be fairly fine to make pecan balls. Put the ground pecans in a mixing bowl. Add the chocolate mixture and stir well. This mixture needs to stay in the fridge until it is no longer sticky. This may take 1 or 2 hours or longer. Stir now and then. Before you shape the balls, stir one egg white into the nuts. This will make the balls hang together for easier shaping. If you use a fresh egg white, add 1 teaspoon of water to it and beat well for a moment. If you use sterilized egg white, use 3 tablespoons. Form large grape–sized balls and put them on a tray or cookie sheet to dry. You should get four pecan balls to the ounce. You do not have to form balls; at Easter time, shape some eggs, if you like. The total yield for this recipe is 17 ounces of candy. One ounce has 5.4 grams of carb and 1.4 grams of protein. The nuts have 3.3 grams of protein per ounce. Weigh the candy to be sure.

Variation: White or Bittersweet Pecan Balls

You can substitute white or bittersweet chocolate for the milk chocolate. Use the same amounts of chocolate. Directions and nutrition counts remain the same.

Variation: Macadamia or Other Nut Balls

For a little variety, alter the nuts in the candy. Make macadamia nut candy and surprise friends on the low-carb diet. You can use walnuts, hazelnuts, or almonds. There is a slight variation in carb counts, but it's not significant.

Sublime Truffles

If you want to bite into a creamy, voluptuous, normally forbidden truffle, make some of these. Keep a few in your fridge (they keep for about 10 days) and freeze the rest. Even if you normally prefer milk chocolate, you may get slightly more chocolate flavor out of semisweet chocolate. The chocolate is only a small part of the recipe, so the distinction between milk chocolate and dark chocolate dissipates a bit, anyway. The taste of the chocolate, however, makes a difference. Try several varieties until you find the one you like best.

PREPARATION TIME: 30 minutes. (The truffle compound needs to harden in the fridge for several hours or overnight before shaping into truffles.)

SERVING SIZE: 1 truffle. AMOUNT PER SERVING: 1.4 grams of carb, 0.4 gram of protein. NUMBER OF SERVINGS: 64.

		CHO (g)	PRO (g)
TRUFFLES			
3	ounces chocolate of your choice	54.0	8.8
5	ounces cream cheese	4.0	10.5
8	tablespoons butter (1 stick)	0	0
½	cup heavy cream	3.2	2.4
2	teaspoons vanilla extract	1.0	0
	trace of salt (shake or two)	0	0
20	packets Splenda sugar substitute	20.0	0
COATING MIX			
2	teaspoons unsweetened cocoa	1.7	0.5
2	teaspoons sugar	8.0	0
	Total	*91.9*	*21.7*

Make the truffles by putting all of the ingredients in the top of a double boiler over hot, not boiling, water. Stir the mixture occasionally as it melts. Toward the end, use a wire whisk to get the mixture totally smooth. Remove from heat. Cool. Put the truffle mixture in the fridge and allow it to harden; this takes at least a few hours.

For the coating mix, combine the cocoa and sugar in a small bowl. Take the truffle compound from the fridge. Work fast. Shape the truffles with a teaspoon into the size of grapes. Drop a few in the coating mix and shake to coat. Shape the balls a final time and set the finished truffles on a plate. If the truffle mixture gets too soft while you are working with it, return it to the fridge for a bit. You can also take out half the amount in the beginning and leave the rest refrigerated. Put candy in small individual paper cups and store in a closed container in the fridge or freezer.

Chocolate Hazelnut Spread

It is a delicious spread, adored by kids and adults alike—but ordinarily impossible to justify on a low-carb diet. Enjoy.

PREPARATION TIME: 20 minutes.

SERVING SIZE: 1 tablespoon. AMOUNT PER SERVING: 1.3 grams of carb, 0.7 gram of protein. NUMBER OF SERVINGS: 76.

		CHO (gm)	PRO (gm)
2	ounces milk chocolate	36.0	7.0
2	ounces unsweetened chocolate bars	8.0	5.8
10	ounces butter (1 stick plus		
	2 tablespoons)	0	0
2	cups heavy cream	12.8	9.6
2	teaspoons vanilla extract	1.0	0
20	packets Splenda sugar substitute	20.0	0
	trace of salt (shake or two)	0	0
2	cups ground hazelnuts	21.6	29.6
	Total	*99.4*	*49.0*

Preheat oven to 300°F or 325°F. Put hazelnuts in a shallow baking pan—you can roast a larger amount if you like—and roast for about 20 to 30 minutes. Check early. Do not let them brown even slightly. Cool. You can prepare these nuts at any time and store them until you need them. Grind hazelnuts in a food processor, if possible. This recipe needs a very fine grind.

Put all of the ingredients except for the hazelnuts in the top of a double boiler and melt slowly. Stir the mixture occasionally as it melts. Toward the end, use a wire whisk to get the mixture totally smooth. Remove from heat and stir in the hazelnuts. Divide this mixture into small portions. Freeze all extras. Keeps refrigerated for about 2 weeks. For easier spreading, remove from the fridge about an hour before you want to use it.

DESSERT SAUCES

These sauces are delicious on low-carb cakes and also on what is to follow—ice cream!

Rhubarb Sauce

There are just 3.3 grams of carb per cup of raw (fresh), diced rhubarb. It's great with all of the crepes, pancakes, waffles, and much more in this cookbook. Make it thick and it can double as jam for the tasty breads, rolls, muffins, and crackers you'll be making. Thin it down and it becomes a syrup. If you have the freezer space, you might want to prepare rhubarb sauce ahead for the winter months (multiply the recipe for larger amounts). It is most practical to start out with a concentrated sauce and thin it as desired.

PREPARATION TIME: 10 minutes. COOKING TIME: 15 to 25 minutes. SERVING SIZE: 1 tablespoon. AMOUNT PER SERVING: 0.4 gram of carb, no protein. NUMBER OF SERVINGS: 32.

		CHO (g)	PRO (g)
4	cups raw, chopped rhubarb	13.2	0
1	lemon slice	1.0	0
	Total	*14.2*	*0*

Place the rhubarb and lemon in a heavy saucepan with 1¼ cups water. Heat and allow to simmer slowly. The rhubarb should get soft but not mushy. Rhubarb at the bottom tends to cook much faster, so stir fairly often. Small amounts of rhubarb cook within a matter of minutes. Cool. Measure sauce. You should have 2 cups. If needed, add water to make up any deficit; stir. Divide the sauce in desired portions and freeze whatever you do not intend to use within a week. Sweeten with Splenda only the amounts you are ready to use and count the extra carb grams. Thin the sauce as desired. A tablespoon of thick sauce makes a great "jam" for a roll or a slice of bread.

Variation: Cranberry Sauce

Follow the directions for making rhubarb sauce (above), but substitute 1 12-ounce package of cranberries, fresh or frozen (28.0 grams of carb). Use 1½ cups of water. Cover and simmer cranberries very slowly for 60 to 90 minutes (longer than simmering rhubarb). Remove lemon. Cool. You should have 2 cups of concentrated cranberry sauce at 0.9 gram of carb per tablespoon. (If needed, add water to make up 2 cups.)

Blueberry Sauce

This sauce is quick to make. You can use fresh or frozen berries, so you can make it at any time during the year. Serve blueberry sauce over the pancake, waffle, cheesecake, and custard recipes in this book; you will find many other delicious uses. Cook the sauce without added sweetener and sweeten whatever portion you are using. A little bit of eggplant added to the blueberries helps thicken it without spoiling the texture or flavor. The sauce keeps for a few days in the fridge but also can be frozen.

PREPARATION TIME: 20 minutes. COOKING TIME: 12 minutes.
SERVING SIZE: 1 tablespoon. AMOUNT PER SERVING: 1.0 gram of carb, negligible amount of protein. NUMBER OF SERVINGS: 40.

		CHO (g)	PRO (g)
2	cups fresh or frozen blueberries	32.4	1.0
2	tablespoons lemon juice	2.6	0
4	ounces peeled and cubed eggplant	4.0	1.1
	Total	*39.0*	*2.1*

Put all of the ingredients in a heavy saucepan with 1 cup water and simmer for about 12 minutes on low. Put the sauce in a food processor or blender and mix briefly so that the sauce still retains some texture. (If you have neither appliance, use a potato masher.) Measure the sauce. You should have at least 2½ cups. (If needed, add water; if you want to make the sauce a little thinner, add enough water to make 3 cups and save another 0.1 gram of carb per tablespoon.) Refrigerate until ready to use. Serve cold or hot. Add Splenda as desired. Count any added carb grams.

Variation: Uncooked Blueberry Sauce

Follow the recipe for Blueberry Sauce (above) but reduce water to ½ cup. Eliminate the eggplant. Mix in a blender or food processor. Keep refrigerated. Measure the resulting liquid. Total carb grams are 35.0. If the total is 1½ cups, 1 tablespoon has 1.6 grams of carb before adding Splenda.

Vanilla Ice Cream

This legendary dessert is loved by almost everyone. Buying commercial ice cream, though, is not easy on a low-carb diet. Low- or no-sugar ice creams invariably seem to be wedded to low-fat creams, too. Richer ice creams come loaded with sugar. So you've got to do it yourself, as usual. Luckily, it is really easy to do—if you have an ice-cream maker. You can make good ice cream from even an inexpensive ice-cream maker. All you do is add the ice-cream mixture, turn it on, and in about 20 minutes you have ice cream. It's yummy. A commercial treat like this runs between 18.0 and 32.0 grams of carb per $\frac{1}{2}$ cup.

PREPARATION TIME: 15 to 20 minutes.

SERVING SIZE: $\frac{1}{2}$ cup. AMOUNT PER SERVING: 4.5 grams of carb, 3.5 grams of protein. NUMBER OF SERVINGS: 6.

		CHO (g)	PRO (g)
2	cups light cream*	12.8	9.6
$\frac{1}{2}$	cup water	0	0
2	teaspoons vanilla extract	1.0	0
12	packets Splenda sugar substitute	12.0	0
4	egg yolks	1.2	11.2
	Total	*27.0*	*20.8*

Slowly heat 1 cup cream, Splenda sugar substitute, and vanilla extract in the top part of a double boiler over hot but not boiling water. Stir or whisk occasionally.

Put the egg yolks in a heavy glass jar and beat until smooth. As the cream begins to heat, dribble a little of it (about 1 tablespoon or so at a time) into the yolks, constantly beating the yolks as you do. Repeat this with about half of the cream. Add the egg yolks and cream to the double boiler. Whisk mixture constantly until it thickens and coats a spoon (in a minute or so). Take double boiler from heat and whisk in the remaining $\frac{1}{2}$ cup cold cream and $\frac{1}{2}$ cup water. You can strain the mixture through a sieve if you like. Put the custard in a bowl and refrigerate, covered, for 2 hours or longer. Ice cream tastes best freshly made. If you want it for dessert, make it close to that time. Follow the directions supplied by the manufacturer. You can also turn this ice cream into great popsicles.

---

* You can substitute 2½ cups of half and half for the combined cream and water. This adds a total of 13.2 grams of carb and 18 grams of protein. A serving has 6.7 grams of carb and 6.4 grams of protein.

Variation: Lemon Ice Cream

Reduce water to ¼ cup. Stir ¼ cup lemon juice into the custard when you take it off the heat. Increase the packets of Splenda to 18. Total carb grams rise to 38.2 grams. The total yield is about 6¼ cups. A ½ cup serving has 6.4 grams of carb.

Variation: Chocolate Ice Cream

Add 1½ ounces of unsweetened chocolate (6.0 grams of carb) to the custard when it is being stirred in the double boiler; do this before the egg yolks have been added. Stir until dissolved. Increase the packets of Splenda to 18. Check for sweetness. The total carb grams are 39.0. The protein change is insignificant. The total yield is about 3½ cups. There are 5.6 grams of carb in ½ cup.

Variation: Raspberry Ice Cream

Use 1½ cups of fresh raspberries. This adds 8.9 grams of carb. Put the berries in a blender or food processor and crush them to a smooth puree or leave them chunky, whichever you like. Add the berries to the custard when it is completed, at the same time you add the remaining cream. Stir. You may need to increase the Splenda, but taste the ice cream first. This recipe yields about 4 cups. Without added sweetener, each serving has 4.5 grams of carb.

Variation: Vanilla-Flavored Milk Shake

In a blender, mix ½ cup Vanilla Ice Cream with ½ cup whipping cream and ½ cup water. Add 2 packets of Splenda (or to taste) and 1 teaspoon vanilla extract. This makes a 12-ounce vanilla milk shake. Total carb grams are 11.0. Protein is 7.0 grams.

Variation: Chocolate-Flavored Milk Shake

In a blender, mix ½ cup Chocolate Ice Cream with ½ cup whipping cream and ½ cup water. Add 2 packets of Splenda (or to taste) and 1 teaspoon vanilla extract. This makes a 12-ounce chocolate milk shake. Total carb grams are 12.5. Protein is 7.5 grams.

Variation: Strawberry (or Other Berry) Milk Shake

In a blender, mix ¾ cup ripe strawberries (or other berries) with ½ cup Vanilla Ice Cream and ¼ cup heavy cream. This makes a 12-ounce strawberry milk shake. If needed, add a small amount of water. Total carb grams are 13.4. Protein is 7.0 grams.

MAIL-ORDER SOURCES

FOODS

True Food Markets
1289 W. 635 South
Orem, UT 84058
Phone: 877-274-5914
Fax: 801-426-7627
Email: support@truefoodsmarket.com

This company has many products you need at very reasonable prices, competitive with those at Vitamin Cottage (below). They have vital wheat gluten flour and just about any nuts you might want. They are a source for whole almond meal, blanched almond meal, and also for a very finely ground blanched almond flour.

Vitamin Cottage—Natural Food Markets
12612 Alameda Parkway
Lakewood, CO 80228
Phone: 303-986-4600
Fax: 303-986-1891
Email: mailorder@vitamincottage.com

Vitamin Cottage is an excellent source of virtually all foods you need for low-carb baking and cooking. Prices appear to be extremely reasonable for all items (but you might want to do your own checking and price comparisons). If you order in bulk, you get better prices yet. On orders over $100, you pay no shipping charge (or a reduced charge if the items are heavy). Items you may want to buy from them are whole almond meal; vital wheat gluten flour; whey protein powder; soy protein powder; soy flours; whole almonds and other nuts. They do not carry almond meal made from blanched almonds. (For a source of blanched almond meal, see Bob's Red Mill.) The Vitamin Cottage carries sweeteners, including sugar alcohols and Stevia, but no Splenda products.

Bob's Red Mill Natural Foods, Inc.
5209 S.E. International Way
Milwaukee, OR 97222
Phone: 800-349-2173
Fax: 503-653-1339
www.bobsredmill.com

You can ask them for a catalog. The blanched, ground almonds are simply called almond meal. (The Mill does not carry whole almond meal.)

COSTCO
www.costco.com

If you are a member, you may be able to purchase the packet form of Splenda sugar substitute at very reasonable prices (in bulk). COSTCO is also a good source for whole almonds, pecans, and walnuts year-round.

New West Foods
5800 Franklin Street
Denver, CO 80216
Phone: 888-NEW-WEST (888-639-9378)
Fax: 303-831-1292
www.NewWestFoods.com

Purveyors of wild game, buffalo, and ostrich. Their products are available in many grocery stores nationwide or by delivery from the company.

Lasater Grasslands Beef, LLC
Matheson, CO
Phone: 866-4LG-BEEF, within Colorado 719-541-2855
www.lasatergrasslandsbeef.com
Purveyors of grass-fed, free-range natural beef products.

For purveyors of natural beef products in or near your state, as well as a wealth of information about the benefits of eating natural beef, check out www.eatwild.com.

La Tortilla Factory
Santa Rosa, CA
Phone: 800-446-1516
www.latortillafactory.com
Purveyors of ready-made low-carb tortillas and burrito wraps.

KITCHEN EQUIPMENT

Precision Weighing Balances
10 Peabody Street
Bradford, MA 01835-7614
Phone: 978-521-7095
Fax: 978-374-5568
Email: sales@balances.com

This company sells commercial-type scales but also small precision scales for weighing 2,000 grams or less. They are accurate and you can reset the scales. Before you purchase, check out scales in kitchen supply stores.

Chef's
P.O. Box 620048
Dallas, TX 75262-0048
Phone: 800-338-3232
Fax: 800-967-3291
www.chefscatalog.com

A good source for hard-to-find items such as a 10-inch griddle (for making crepes) and taco racks. Ask for a catalog.

Chicago Metallic: The Bakeware Company
800 Ela Road
Lake Zurich, IL 60047
Phone: 888-391-2020
www.bakingpans.com

This company makes heavy-weight metal bakeware that is ideal for baking with the low-carb products in this cookbook. Their products are available in many stores nationwide. Check out their website to see what is available and to get more information.

HEALTH REPORT

For a free sample issue of the *Eades Health Report* newsletter, write to Editor, Eades Health Report, P.O. Box 62, Denver, CO 80201, or click on www.eadeshealthreport.com, where you'll find up-to-date nutritional and health information. Also visit the Drs. Eades' web site at www.eatprotein.com for information about available nutritional products or for dietary support.

Also available wherever books are sold:

The 30-Day Low-Carb Diet Solution
By Michael R. Eades, M.D., and Mary Dan Eades, M.D.

- Maximum results with minimum fuss
- High-protein recipes that stop your cravings
- Customized meal plans

from Wiley
ISBN 0-471-43050-1

INDEX